For more information, contact us at:

The Council on Aging of Greater Nashville
95 White Bridge Road, Suite 114
Nashville, TN 37205

Info@councilonaging-midtn.org

Visit our website at:
www.councilonaging-midtn.org

ISBN 10:   0-9818184-8-x

ISBN 13:   978-0-9818184-8-1

Edited by Ted Griffith

Cover Design by Carlo da Silva

Interior Design by Katherine Goodman

Compliments of
The Tennessee Conference of
The United Methodist Church
Health and Welfare Committee
2012

Contents

  - General Resource List
  - Financial Records Inventories
  - Insurance Inventories
  - Legal Documents Inventory
  - Medication Record Forms
  - Glossary of Medical Conditions
  - Glossary of Medical Tests, Therapies, and Procedures
  - Future Caregiving Checklist
  - Questions to Ask When Hiring a Private Care Service
  - Recipes for Additional Nutrition

Preface

> *Let us take care of the children, for they have a long way to go.*
> *Let us take care of the elders, for they have come a long way.*
> *Let us take care of those in between, for they are doing the work.*
>
> ~ African Proverb

This book is addressed to all concerned caregivers – daughters, sons, spouses, grandchildren, siblings, best friends, and neighbors. The majority of the caregivers in this country do seem to be women, and we are grateful for initial funding from the Women's Fund of the Community Foundation of Middle Tennessee, Gannett Foundation, West End Home Foundation, and Tennessee State University Center for Aging Social Work Program. Production of the second edition was begun with donations made to the Council on Aging of Greater Nashville in memory of Elizabeth Gwinn, the mother of one of the committee members.

This book is written with our local community in mind, but the issues addressed and services available are provided in different ways nationwide. Local senior centers, Area Agency on Aging and Disability offices, the Eldercare Locator (800-677-1116), and a variety of websites can identify what is available elsewhere.

COMMITTEE – AGING & CARING: THINGS FAMILIES NEED TO KNOW

Council on Aging thanks the following professionals, seniors and caregivers (sometimes all three in the same person) who worked to compile this resource book:

Clenna Ashley — Banker, Lawyer, Caregiver
Caroline Chamberlain — Council on Aging of Greater Nashville, caregiver
Amanda Chiavini — Graduate Student, Vanderbilt University
Beth Dunlap — Registered Dietitian, Simply Healthy
Maribeth Farringer — Council on Aging of Greater Nashville, caregiver
Barbara Heflin — GNRC Area Agency on Aging & Disability
Jennifer Kim — Vanderbilt University School of Nursing
Suzanne Lanier — Elder Resource Consultants
Betty C. Moore — Council on Aging of Greater Nashville
Elizabeth Moss — WholeCare Connections
Diane Schlaufman — GNRC Area Agency on Aging & Disability
Grace S. Smith — Council on Aging of Greater Nashville
Gwen Smith — Council on Aging of Greater Nashville
Lee Stewart — Metro Social Services
Jane Stumpf — Caregiver
Jean Stumpf — Council on Aging of Greater Nashville
Kelly Tipler — Tennessee Respite Coalition

The following individuals contributed to the initial publication:

Nell Clark, Margaret Dye, Jennifer Ferguson, Nancy Fletcher, Phyllis Frank, Ann Harwell, Annette Hutchinson, Margie Ward Johnson, Linda Varnell.

Special thanks for assistance in preparing and editing this publication:

Ted Griffith

Introduction

Are you worried about an elderly relative or friend? Is he or she moving more slowly, eating less, or forgetting things? Is this normal aging, or are there things that need attention? Is he or she denying that anything is wrong, or is he or she aware of problems, perhaps worried and waiting for some help from you? Of course, if there is a major event such as a stroke, heart attack, or serious fall, you are suddenly aware of a need but maybe uncertain of how best to help.

Each family has its own history and dynamics. However, the basic issue common to all is how family members can be helpful and still preserve the dignity and as much independence as possible for an aging person. The family often wants to rush in to help, and while well meaning, they may overwhelm a slower-thinking or moving older adult. Sometimes it is hard for a child to face the deterioration of a parent. Many times siblings disagree on what can or should be done, or a well senior may have different ideas about the care of an aging spouse. The reality is that they each bring something different and important to the table, and they all need each other.

If possible, planning ahead as a family is the best way to approach this part of the family's future. This book provides guidelines for issues to be addressed and options that may be workable for all concerned.

A first step can be to talk with the person needing care about his/her expectations for the future, without making assumptions. A useful technique is to focus your concerns and questions on yourself ("I'm feeling concerned that you might fall coming down the stairs").

Many seniors face their aging concerns realistically and make many of their own plans as a "gift to their family." This book can help these seniors identify those issues and consider the options. Planning ahead for the aging process has many unknowns, because the exact nature of individual aging issues is not predictable. Still, there are many concrete steps that can be taken to ease the aging process as it evolves.

For the purpose of this book, "family" is defined as whoever makes up the relationship between elder and caregiver. This can include friends and neighbors as well as blood relatives.

COUNCIL ON
AGING

Organizing
and
Planning Ahead:
A Gift to You
and to Your Family

And so the journey begins ...

When one widow began to experience short-term memory loss that interfered with her ability to function alone, her greatest gift to her three daughters was to seek their support in what was to become, as Nancy Reagan wrote, "a long goodbye." She had a choice: to "go it alone" as long as she could and isolate herself from those who loved her most; or to draw them into her world while she was still able, allowing all to share in a tapestry of memories, tears, laughter, and love that would forever enrich their lives.

After a diagnosis of depression transitioned into one of Alzheimer's, the widow first became very practical with her daughters. Plans were necessary, but decisions were almost impossible to make alone. Each family member played a unique role, according to her abilities and her desires. Was the road easy? No. Were there times of deep soul-searching and honest conversations? Yes. Was there conflict? Some ... but less than expected. Husbands also played a strong supporting role but remained in the background – more as support for their wives and sisters-in-law. Did they make mistakes? Of course! However, they were determined to muddle through, to lean on their God, to communicate honestly, and to love one another unconditionally.

The journey began with wills, powers of attorney, difficult, and endless conversations on end-of-life issues such as tube feeding, do not resuscitate orders (DNR), funeral wishes, etc. Resolving all issues was a process over a year's time.

... continued next page

As their mother's world began to change and her environment needed to change, they all had to address the matter of "things"! She would select items of equal value and set them aside until her family was gathered. They would draw cards with numbers that corresponded to numbers on the items. Matched numbers meant the item was theirs. After a draw, some real horse-trading would go on – laughter, memories, and some tears ... but a deep sense of family heritage. It gave the mother joy to be able to share and actively direct this giving, which would continue at her direction over the years as her world became smaller and smaller and her needs changed.

Now, as her journey here is ending, she has planned so that her family can care for her without the worry of financial burdens, funeral arrangements, disbursement of property, etc. They are able, within the plan she set forth, to be flexible in meeting her spiritual, emotional, and physical needs.

Crisis, or sometimes even planning for crisis, can bring to the surface all past losses with parent/sibling or sibling/sibling relationships. It might be wise to use a facilitator outside the family to lead or direct this process. This might be a healthcare professional skilled in this area, a hospital social worker or discharge planner, a psychologist or a psychiatrist, or an attorney who specializes in mediation to specifically help families in dealing with aging issues. Some financial planners also offer this service. Several community agencies listed in this publication can also provide ready resources or links to community resources that assist families in this process.

Family Meeting

In planning a family conference, consider including those who live far away and those who are extended family members. The most important attendee is the senior. If the senior senses that there are decisions being made or considered without his/her input, feelings of anger, isolation, anxiety, helplessness, and depression may emerge. The senior has the legal and moral right to make his/her own decisions and to participate in plans affecting his/her life. A person's desires and decisions should only be questioned when there is brain deterioration or his/her decisions are endangering his/her life or the lives of others. If the elder is unable to attend, keep him/her informed and involved in the decisions made.

What is discussed in a family conference? The spouse, adult children, and other important relatives and friends collectively talk about what their elder can reasonably expect and accept from them. Early sessions can be stormy, and old conflicts and slights can surface. Invitations to elders should be carefully phrased. (e.g., "Mom, there is some planning that we can do now that will give us more choices and options later.")

PREPARING

- Before the meeting an effort should be made to gather as much information about the elder's condition and situation as possible.

- Most elderly want to maintain their independence as long as possible. Be balanced and sensitive in your approach. It is important to not move too fast.

■ The sooner a family conference takes place, the better it is for your senior and the family. It gives an opportunity to avoid misunderstandings, to recognize and assign responsibilities, and to consider options that reflect the parent's preferences and feelings.

■ While one meeting is good, periodic meetings are best.

PURPOSE / GOALS

■ To learn your senior's preferences, wishes, and feelings about housing, health, finances, insurance, legal documents, crisis care, long-term care, and end-of-life issues.

■ To determine, as permitted by the senior, the current state of his/her legal and financial affairs.

■ To identify available resources to enrich your elder spiritually, physically, socially, intellectually, and emotionally.

■ To help your elder make decisions about his/her affairs, future, and crisis and long-term care.

■ To help your elder maintain the level of control he/ she wishes and that is feasible, while hearing his/her concerns and fears as well as those of other family members.

SUGGESTED AGENDA

■ Designate someone to take notes.

Complete/organize the following:

■ **Personal Information**

This comprises what many services refer to as "the face sheet" and is the information almost every entity will ask for before providing information or service. Examples are Social Security, Medicare, and Insurance Policy numbers, names of doctors, and all prescription and non-prescription medications. Have this information handy when calls are made.

■ **Legal Information** (See Financial and Legal Chapter)

Your elder may not be ready to divulge this information. Encourage him/her to make an appointment with his/her attorney to complete the documents. The important thing is that all have been collected and that you know the location of all documents.

■ **Medical Information** (See Negotiating the Healthcare System Chapter)

Your elder should bring a sack containing all medications, any printouts from physicians, and his/her address book or phone book containing phone numbers and addresses of medical professionals.

■ **Financial Information** (See Financial and Legal Chapter)

Your elder may not be ready to divulge this information. Encourage the senior to make an appointment with his/her CPA or financial planner to complete the documents. The important thing is that all have been collected and you know the location of all documents.

■ **Insurance Information** (See Financial and Legal Chapter)

Make a copy of insurance cards. Look for overlapping or unnecessary policies. Know location of policies.

THINKING AHEAD

After you've established your plan and sorted out who will do what, you will need to be flexible about adjusting it. What works today may not work well next year or next month. Do your best to anticipate your elder's needs and address concerns proactively. When it comes to looking after your elder, you always have to be on the ball. There's no doubt that the balancing act is exhausting. But, ultimately, it's one that your elder will appreciate and that you will find rewarding.

Family Meeting "Dos" and "Don'ts"

DO

☑ Listen to your elder's feelings of frustration and/or dependency as he/she reacts to life changes. Acknowledge the losses/changes the senior is facing.

☑ Focus on your elder's strengths and abilities while considering his/her limitations.

☑ Make "I" statements. (e.g., "I realize this must be overwhelming. I can only imagine how you must be feeling ..." or "I know you must be sad ...").

☑ Assess the resources and knowledge of various family members. Remember that each family member has a unique relationship with the elder and with each other. Consider if any of the changes are being contemplated in order to make you or your family member feel more comfortable without regard to your elder's feelings or wishes.

☑ Consider spouses and children when making decisions. They should be a part of making decisions that affect them, and their needs, fears and limitations should be respected.

DON'T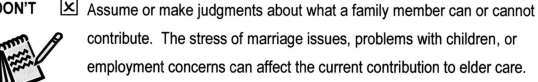

☒ Assume or make judgments about what a family member can or cannot contribute. The stress of marriage issues, problems with children, or employment concerns can affect the current contribution to elder care.

☒ Force your values and fears on your elder; he or she has their own, and it is important for them to continue to practice them.

☒ Make promises (e.g., "We will never put you in a nursing home."). Circumstances may eventually prevent you from keeping your promise, fostering guilt for you and mistrust from your elder.

☒ Assume tasks or functions that your senior can do, even with some difficulty. Your elder will resent forced dependency or will become even more dependent (accelerating depression). Everyone needs to feel a sense of accomplishment and purpose.

☒ Let unresolved feelings regarding your elder or other family members result in inappropriate decisions, such as avoiding the elder or the relative, trying to please at any price, or finding fault with the elder's behavior or with family members' support and care of the elder. Taking heroic measures, without assistance, to care for your elder can seriously impact the total well-being of your spouse, your children, and yourself.

**Adapted from *"Help! Where Are All My Papers?"* and *"Help! Am I the Parent Now?"* by Sheryl Cook and Farrar Moore.

Long Distance Caregiving

Caring From Afar

My Mom lived in Little Rock, Arkansas; I live in the Nashville, Tennessee area, and my only sibling lives in Richmond, Virginia. Mom's health began slowly deteriorating. Each visit, I noticed she was doing less and she began having falls. She wanted me and my sister, DeAnn, to think she was okay. When we visited, she made a great effort to show us she was taking care of herself. DeAnn had the foresight to get Mom to sign a Power of Attorney, get Life Alert and talked to her about selling her house.

After one particularly bad fall, Mom's friends let us know exactly what was going on with her. They had been doing the caregiving and couldn't take care of her and themselves anymore. I found a realtor who had been through a similar situation with her Mom. A personal support service agency put us in touch with a housing referral service geared toward seniors. They gave us options for Mom, plus emotional support. We got Mom to agree to sell her house and move to a retirement center near me in Nashville.

DeAnn and I spent a week with Mom sorting through 50+ years worth of stuff. We laughed and cried. It was very bittersweet. Mom's not been happy about the move. It's not been easy on any of us. But it was the best decision for all of us. We know for certain that Mom is safe and getting the care she needs.

-- *Terri Humel*

The logistical burden of coordinating someone's care from afar, with all the phone calls and visits home, can be incredibly time-consuming. It can also affect work performance. The initial process of planning and organizing is the same as in any caregiving situation and is vitally important.

Long distance caregivers face the inconvenience and high price of traveling to and from their elder's home base. But perhaps the biggest obstacle long distance caregivers must overcome is the guilt of not being there all the time. When you are able to make a visit, find ways to make each visit rich and meaningful, perhaps by connecting with old friends and family members.

Of course, not all long distance caregivers can drop everything and move. What's important is establishing a nearby support network for your elders--whether it's composed of relatives or friends and neighbors. Most areas also have websites that are helpful. Look for Area Agencies on Aging, disease support agencies (e.g., Alzheimer's or Diabetes Associations), or free online referral services with access to professionals who can assist with assessments and resources. There are services that provide supervision when family members are not around. The National Association of Geriatric Care Managers has members in many communities.

For assistance in arranging a move, Senior Move Managers can do much of the hands-on work for a fee. These professionals can prepare a house for sale, pack up furnishings, help the senior determine what to give away or sell, and fully set up the new home.

When you visit your loved one, ask him/her or ask friends in the community about resources known to be good and reliable. Area hospitals or your loved one's local physicians may also be good resources. If applicable, make contact with the place where your elder worships, and be sure the congregation knows how to reach you. Ask about support ministries and activities available there. Identify three resources of support in your elder's city and have their contact numbers/addresses. Be sure the support resources have your contact information and can easily reach you. Maintain and nurture these associations in an open and honest way that is not patronizing or humiliating to your elder.

Talk to your employer or Human Resource Department. Caring for elderly relatives is becoming more common. You may be surprised at some resources available and/or the flexibility that your company may offer you.

If there are good support systems of friends and neighbors and no serious health problems, it is advisable for an elder to stay where he/she has been living. When serious health problems develop, the need for a facility near family members may be needed. This enables the family to visit and to more readily supervise care.

Resources

- *Help! Where Are All My Papers?*
  - Sheryl Cook and Farrar Moore

- *The Dying Time*
  - Joan Furman

- *And Thou Shalt Honor, The Caregiver's Companion*
  - edited by Beth Witrogen McLeod

- *Aging With Grace*
  - David Snowden, PhD

- *The 36-Hour Day*
  - Nancy L. Mace and Peter V. Rabins, M.D., M.P.H.

- *The Fearless Caregiver*
  - Gary Barg

- *Helping Yourself Help Others: A Book for Caregivers*
  - Rosalynn Carter and Susan K. Golant

- *Caring for Your Aging Parent When Love Is Not Enough*
  - Barbara Deane

- *The Art of Forgiving*
  - Lewis Smedes

- *Getting Through the Night*
  - Eugenia Price

- *I Love You But You Drive Me Crazy: A Guide for Caring Relatives*
  - Calder and Watt

- *The Magic of Humor in Caregiving: Preventing Caregiver Burnout*
  - James R. Sherman, PhD

- *Please Take Me Home Before Dark: One Family's Journey with Alzheimer's Disease*
  - Billie J. Pate & Mary Pate Yarnell

- *Living Fully, Dying Well*
  - Reuben Job 2007—United Methodist Resources

There are many other good resources from the National Institute on Aging and other such organizations that can be located online.

PERIODICALS

- *Today's Caregiver*
- *The Healthy Caregiver*
- *The Magazine for Adult Children of Aging Parents*
- *Wiser Now*
- *Alzheimer's Disease Caregiver Tips*

HELPFUL WEBSITES

- http://www.aarp.org

  Formerly known as the American Association of Retired Persons, AARP is a United States-based non-governmental, non-profit, non-partisan membership organization for people aged 50 and over, dedicated to enhancing quality of life with age.

- http://www.eldercare.gov

  The United States' Health and Human Services Department which provides local information, referral resources, and contact information for state and local agencies,.

- http://www.caregiver.org

  Offering programs at national, state and local levels to support and sustain caregivers, Family Caregiver Alliance was the first community-based non-profit organization in the country to address the needs of families and friends providing long-term care at home.

■ http://www.caregiving.org

Focusing on issues of family caregiving, the National Alliance for
Caregiving is a non-profit coalition of national organizations. Alliance
members include grassroots organizations, professional associations,
service organizations, disease-specific organizations, a government
agency, and corporations.

■ http://www.caremanager.org

Professional Geriatric Care Managers (PGCMs) are health and human
services specialists who help families care for older relatives, while
encouraging as much independence as possible. The PGCM acts as a
guide and advocate in identifying problems and offering solutions,
from assessment of an aging parent's needs to addressing the life
change of a family affected by Alzheimer's Disease, Parkinson's, or
other symptoms of dementia.

COUNCIL ON
AGING

Financial and Legal Issues
and
Medical Insurance

Financial affairs are often one of the first areas where your elder needs a helping hand.

Unopened Mail Equals Trouble

Betty noticed that the table where the mail was kept was getting higher and higher each time she visited. If she sat with her mother and went through the papers, she often found late notices for unpaid utilities, new credit cards, and insurance terminations for non-payment. It was clear that some help was needed. Betty and her mother Sarah arranged to spend time every week going through the mail. Betty would write the checks that were due, and her mother signed them. This helped Sarah feel that she still had control over her money and how it was spent and helped Betty feel confident that important bills were being paid. They also discussed the dangers of accepting new credit card offers and Sarah's discussing financial affairs with telemarketers, who often called in the evening, when Sarah was lonely and eager to talk. Betty added Sarah's telephone number to the national and state Do Not Call List to help cut down on the number of telemarketing calls. Eventually, Sarah and Betty went to the bank and signed new signature cards so that Betty could sign checks and withdraw money from Sarah's bank accounts.

The first step to financial and legal organization is often a review of important documents. This is a brief list of documents which might be needed. They should be located and updated, as the needs of the senior change.

FINANCIAL RECORDS INVENTORY
(See Resources and Inventories Chapter for copies of forms)

A. All **bank accounts** with the account numbers and who is authorized to sign. **Certificates of Deposit** and interest rates and due dates should be noted. **Safe Deposit Box** contents should be listed and renewal date noted. The location of the safe deposit key is very important. If the key is lost, it will take time and money to have the box drilled so that the contents can be accessed. Some bank accounts can be set up to be payable on death to someone named by the owner, and if this is the sole asset of an estate, can eliminate the need to probate a will. This account type can also be used to leave money to someone, regardless of what a will may state. In most instances joint accounts or payable on death accounts will become the property of the joint owner or named beneficiary, regardless of the terms of any will. There may also be automatic deductions and deposits that should be identified.

B. **Life insurance policies** with the insurance company name, type of policy, policy number, and beneficiaries. Also, list the due date of any payments.

C. **Investments**. This would include brokerage accounts and account numbers, location of any stock certificates held by the senior, location and type of ownership of all real estate, and details of any mortgages.

D. **Income tax returns** for at least three years. These are also useful to find details of investments such as dividends and interest, limited partnerships, and any interest paid on real estate loans.

E. **Military Service Discharge Papers** (DD214) needed to determine Veteran's benefits and to receive American flag for funeral.

F. **Marriage License** needed to file for Social Security using spouse's benefits.

G. **Automobile titles** or **registration** and details of any loans outstanding that are secured by autos.

H. All **property insurance policies** with the insurance company name, type of policy, policy limits, and due dates for premiums.

I. All **health insurance, Medicare Part D,** and **long-term care policies** with the insurance company name, types and amounts of coverage, and due dates for premium payments.

J. **Burial insurance** and **prepaid funeral plans:** Locate cemetery plots and determine the wishes of the senior regarding the funeral, burial or cremation, and whether any expenses have been prepaid. If a spouse has died, a joint headstone may have been purchased, along with a burial plot. If the prepaid funeral plan is irrevocable, it may not count as an asset for Medicaid purposes.

K. **Death certificate** of predeceased spouse.

LEGAL CAPACITY

Legal Capacity is the term used to denote the level of judgment and decision-making ability needed to sign official documents. The requirements for legal capacity may vary from one legal document or proceeding to another. This is an especially important issue for caregivers of those with dementia. If the person with dementia is able to understand the meaning, the importance, and the consequences of a given legal document, he or she likely has the legal capacity to execute or carry out the signing of the document. It may be necessary to ask for medical advice from the senior's physician in determining a person's level of mental ability.

LEGAL DOCUMENTS INVENTORY

(See Resources and Inventories Chapter for copies of forms)

A. **Last Will and Testament**

This document should be reviewed to be certain that it still conveys the wishes of the senior and is current on the property it conveys and the beneficiaries to whom the property is bequeathed. Any special items the senior wishes to leave someone should be listed very specifically. The original will should not be kept in a safe deposit box, as it may be difficult to get into the box, depending on who is authorized, or the bank might not be open. Often the original is kept at a lawyer's office, in which case copies should be made for beneficiaries and/or for those named by the will as Executor or Trustee.

B. Durable Power of Attorney

This document can allow the person named as attorney, often a caregiver, to do anything the senior could do for themselves if they were competent. An attorney familiar with the financial and legal affairs of the senior should draw this up. A Durable Power of Attorney can grant very broad powers or can be limited and may be made effective only upon the mental or physical disability of the senior or the occurrence of certain events. You may have to record the Power of Attorney in the county where the senior resides and obtain certified copies to give to banks, brokerage firms, and others holding assets and to sell any real estate.

C. Power of Attorney for Health Care or Appointment of Health Care Agent

Doctors, hospitals, and other medical agencies will want to know if the senior has a Power of Attorney for Health Care (now called Appointment of Health Care Agent). Copies are often kept in the doctor's records or at a hospital where the senior has previously been cared for. This document allows the person named as attorney to make healthcare decisions for the senior if they are not capable or able to decide for themselves. The person named as the attorney can consent or refuse to consent to treatment, and the power can be subject to any limitations the senior wishes to have included. An Appointment of Health Care Agent form which complies with Tennessee law can be found at
http://health.state.tn.us/advancedirectives and on the Council on Aging website, www.councilonaging-midtn.org.

D. **Living Will or Advance Care Plan**

This provides direction to physicians and family regarding a person's wishes if he or she becomes terminally ill or permanently unconscious. Very specific directions are provided regarding the withholding or provision of food, water, and other nourishment and regarding organ donation. It is a record of decisions the person has made for him/herself. This form was designed to comply with the law in Tennessee and can be found at http://health.state.tn.us/advancedirectives and on the Council of Aging website, www.councilonaging-midtn.org.

E. **Appointment of Surrogate and Physician Orders for Scope of Treatment (POST)** (This form can also be a *Do Not Resuscitate* form). These forms were developed to record the wishes of the patient in the event that he or she becomes incapable of making such decisions. They also provide a form for a physician to appoint a surrogate (a person who can do the things the patient would do if he/she were able) for a patient, to assist in the health care decisions, when the patient is not able to make them and needs a person to protect his/her interests. The physician-appointed surrogate alone cannot make decisions to withhold artificial nutrition and fluid, but if an independent physician also certifies that the continued nutrition and fluids are merely prolonging the act of dying, then they can be withheld. Family members cannot override a POST that is signed by a patient and physician which contains a Do Not Resuscitate order. More information about these and other forms of advance directives can be found at http://health.state.tn.us/advancedirectives and on the Council on Aging website, www.councilonaging-midtn.org.

NEXT STEPS

When the financial and legal records have been examined, there will be other important issues to address. If the caregiver will pay bills or take care of investments, an authorization or durable power of attorney may have to be filed with every institution where assets are held. It will be necessary to change the address and telephone contact numbers to those of the caregiver. To have access to a safe deposit box, the caregiver's name and signature must be added to the signature card at the bank, and a key obtained.

It will also be important to know the **sources of income** and whether the senior has the ability, and under what conditions, to withdraw funds from any retirement accounts, pensions, or trusts. Some accounts such as an **IRA** (Individual Retirement Account) require that the senior begin to withdraw funds at age 70 ½, but withdrawals may be made without penalty upon disability or reaching the age of 59 ½. Upon the death of a spouse (or former spouse), it is important to determine whether using the spouse's benefits (which are often higher for men who were primary wage earners) might provide more income. These benefits are available to an unmarried widow or widower of a person who worked long enough under Social Security to be eligible for benefits. The unmarried divorced spouse of a worker who dies can get benefits just the same as a widow or widower, provided their marriage lasted ten years or more. Benefits paid to a surviving, divorced spouse do not affect the benefit rates for other survivors getting benefits based on the worker's record.

If the senior owns his/her home and moves to a relative's home or a senior housing unit, it may be better to rent the property than to sell.

Renting often provides more income than can be made from investments although it does mean more work for the caregiver. If the senior is able to live on his/her own but lacks income, a **Reverse Mortgage** or **Equity Line of Credit** can help use the equity in the home to provide for living expenses. Department of Housing and Urban Development-approved counselors can provide more information about those options.

Of course, all income will have income tax consequences, and it is important to check with an accountant or financial advisor in order to

> " ... it is important to check with an accountant or financial advisor ... "

make the best decisions regarding the use of available assets. As the senior's ability to travel, drive, and live life changes, it may be sensible to cancel unnecessary services such as newspapers, magazines, some phone services, car insurance, home insurance, and cell phones.

If the health and fitness of the senior allows, long-term care insurance can help provide the money needed later if he/she becomes unable to work or live alone. Long-term care insurance can be purchased even when the senior is in his/her 70s, but after 70 the policy may be too expensive or medically difficult to obtain.

If the senior should suddenly become unable to take care of him/herself, a caregiver must review the bank statements to see what bills are being paid and to discover sources of income. Automatic deductions may need to be discontinued and automatic deposits may need to be changed.

In the event there is not a **Durable Power of Attorney** when the senior becomes unable to take care of his/her financial and legal affairs, it will be necessary to have the court appoint a **Conservator or Guardian** for the affairs of the senior. This will require a doctor's certification, and the court will appoint an attorney to investigate the situation. If the court appoints a Conservator, Letters of Conservatorship will be issued. The guardian will need several copies of these, as they will have to be presented to banks, brokers, and whenever assets are sold. The Letters of Conservatorship act in the same manner as the Durable Power of Attorney, but the court will require that a bond be posted and will have to approve the sale of certain assets. An annual accounting of all income and disbursements will have to be filed each year along with a plan for taking care of the assets owned by the senior. This will also involve attorney fees and court fees in addition to annual payment of the bond.

A Conservator may be entitled to receive payment for his/her services. It may be that a caregiver will need a salary to help cover the cost of the time and effort he/she will devote to taking care of the assets of the senior. The Court will decide whether the Conservator will be paid, but a caregiver will have to work out an arrangement with the senior and possibly with other relatives. In the case that an interest in a house or other asset of the senior is promised in return for care, <u>this should be carefully put in writing, preferably by an attorney, and always while the senior is still competent</u>.

If you are caring for someone's assets, keep meticulous, detailed records. If you are storing information on a computer, keep backup copies and let others know how they can access the information if you become unavailable. This will protect you and the senior you are caring for.

If possible, the senior and the caregiver should work together as soon as feasible to address finances and legalities. Being aware and prepared will provide a much smoother transition into the future for all concerned.

Medicare

Medicare is a federal government health insurance program that provides medical care and prescription benefits. You become eligible for Medicare when you turn 65 years of age or if you are under the age of 65 and have a disability. Medicare has several parts: Part A (Hospital) and Part B (Medical) and Part D (Prescription drug coverage).

MEDICARE PART A AND B

Medicare Part A covers care in hospitals, skilled nursing facilities, hospice care, and limited health care. Most people do not have to pay for part A and will receive it automatically when they turn 65. Medicare Part B is optional and covers doctors' visits, outpatient services, and other items that are medically necessary. There is a standard premium for people who choose Medicare Part B that is generally deducted from monthly Social Security checks. If one decides not to enroll in Medicare Part B, there may be a penalty if enrolled later. To avoid penalty one must sign up within three months before and three months after one's 65th birthday. When becoming eligible for Medicare, you either choose traditional Medicare or Medicare Advantage Plans that are managed care plans (see below for more on Medicare Advantage Plans).

Persons with low income may qualify to have the state pay the premium. This is called QMB, and the local Department of Human Services office can provide an application. When talking with physicians regarding your Medicare, a question to ask is if the doctor accepts assignment. This means the doctor has agreed to charge no more than the amount Medicare has approved for any given service.

Supplemental (Medigap) Insurance

Supplemental insurance, or Medigap, is a separate insurance policy purchased from a private company that covers the deductibles and copayments that Medicare does not cover. This is popular for individuals who opt for traditional Medicare.

MEDICARE PART D

Medicare Part D provides outpatient prescription drug coverage. Part D is optional but has a built-in penalty if not chosen when eligible. The penalty is one percent per month. Considering there is only one open-enrollment period a year, that one percent can add up. It is recommended, even if you are not on medications at the time you are eligible, that you enroll in a low cost plan as a safety net. You never know if you could benefit from it later. An exception to this recommendation is if the present Supplemental or Medigap Insurance policy covers prescription medications.

When choosing a plan, you can choose a stand-alone plan or a Medicare Advantage Plan (see below). A stand-alone plan will cover a prescription drug benefit separately from the Medicare Part A & B coverage. Most, but not all, drug plans charge a monthly premium that varies by plan. Other costs will vary depending on which drugs you use, which plan you choose, and whether or not you get extra help paying your Part D costs.

Medicare drug plans have a coverage gap (also known as the "donut hole"). A coverage gap means that after you have spent a certain amount of money on your prescription drugs you have to pay 100 percent (out of pocket) of drug costs until you have reached "catastrophic coverage." Once one reaches catastrophic coverage, the drug plan will pay 95 percent of drug costs until the end of the year.

Medicare Advantage Plans

A Medicare Advantage Plan combines Parts A, B, and D into one private insurance plan. You pay one monthly premium for your doctor, hospital, and prescription benefits. To get the best value from your Medicare Advantage plan, you need to stay within the plan's network of providers. If your physician is not in-network, you can either pay extra to see that physician or choose another physician who is in-network. A benefit to Medicare Advantage plans is that they can offer more coverage than original plans. For example, some may cover more preventive care or dental and/or eye care. Another benefit is that some Advantage plans do not have a donut hole for prescription coverage. These plans have a higher premium but could save you in the long run if you expect to have high prescription drug costs.

EXTRA HELP

If your income and assets are limited, you may qualify for extra help paying for your Medicare drug plan's monthly premium, yearly deductible, and prescription copays or coinsurance, including any costs you have in the coverage gap. To find out if you are eligible for extra help, or to apply for extra help, contact the Social Security Administration at 1-800-772-1213. Some individuals will automatically qualify for extra help and will not need to apply (such as those on TennCare). However, these individuals will still need to choose a drug plan that best suits their needs.

CHANGING PLANS

You can only change plans once a year during the open enrollment period. Individuals who are receiving extra help are an exception to this and can change their Part D plans once a month. Open enrollment for Part D is from November 15 to December 31. Apply as close to the November 15 date as possible to allow time for the paperwork to be processed before January 1.

Medicaid for Nursing Home Care

Medicare pays for very little nursing home care, primarily skilled care after a hospital stay. Medicaid does pay for nursing home care for low-income citizens who medically qualify.

A person does not have to sell his/her home to get Medicaid to pay for nursing home care. If a spouse is living at home, Medicaid provides certain financial protections for him or her. There are provisions, however, to keep a person from transferring assets just prior to nursing home placement in order to qualify for Medicaid. The local Department of Human Services accepts applications for Medicaid for Nursing Home Care.

Long Term Care Insurance

Most seniors do not wish to go to a nursing home. Long-term care insurance can help pay for in-home care and assisted living as well as nursing home care that is not covered by Medicare. It is important for you to know if your parent has this insurance, when it was purchased, and just what it covers.

Privacy and HIPAA

Since 2003, under the rules and regulations of the Health Insurance Portability and Accountability Act (HIPAA), access to a patient's medical information has been restricted, requiring patient permission for disclosure. Doctors, hospitals, and other health care providers are required to obtain written acknowledgement that they have given patients notice of their right to privacy. They are also prohibited from disclosing certain information other than "as needed" to carry out treatment, receive payment, and implement health care operations. Most providers have forms allowing the patient to authorize certain persons to receive their health care information. It is important that each health care provider be authorized to discuss the senior's health information with a designated person, particularly where the senior may be incompetent or unable to speak. Otherwise, caregivers may not be able to get the information they need to care for their loved ones properly.

Resources

■ Medicare   1-800-633-4227

  http://www.medicare.gov

■ Tennessee Commission on Aging & Disability   1-877-801-0044
  This is the state health insurance assistance program (SHIP). They can provide information on all aspects of Medicare and other programs for seniors.

■ Inspector General's Fraud Hotline   1-800-447-8477
  Call to report Medicare fraud or abuse by health care providers.

Do Not Call List

The goal of these programs is to eliminate unnecessary and unwanted telemarketing calls. Since seniors are often confined to home, they are often the target of such calls.

■ For the Federal Government visit: http://www.donotcall.gov or call
  1-888-382-1222.   This registration is effective for five years.

■ For the State of Tennessee visit: http://www.state.tn.us/tra and go to
  the 'Do Not Call' link or call 1-877-872-7030.

Advance Directives Forms

Downloadable forms are available on the website of the Council on Aging of Greater Nashville, www.councilonaging-midtn.org.

COUNCIL ON
AGING

Negotiating
the
Healthcare System

Health care today is dramatically different from the health care system that your parent or older loved one encountered as a young adult. Today, we have a highly technical system of care with medical diagnostic and treatment advances that have provided great benefit to extend life and improve quality of life. However, this system has financial costs and requires multiple physician and non-physician health care specialists to provide the care. Health insurance, managed care, and Medicare and Medicaid financing have each played a part in directing the health care delivery system. One of the results has been an often fragmented and confusing system of care.

One of the most important skills a caregiver needs is to be able to communicate effectively with the health care professionals who provide care to the family member. You, as the caregiver, are part of the caregiving "team," and your role is vital in obtaining the best medical care for your loved one. As the person who provides hands-on care, you are more likely to be aware of your loved one's history, symptoms, and concerns. In fact, you may have to learn to read non-verbal cues in order to provide needed information to the health care provider if your family member is no longer able to communicate verbally.

> " Your role is vital in obtaining the best medical care for your loved one. "

- Know and respect your loved one's wishes with regard to health care treatment, procedures, and end-of-life issues.

■ Ask your loved one to designate someone to make health care decisions for him/her in the event he/ she is no longer able to make such decisions. This can be done through an advance directive such as a Power of Attorney for Health Care (now called Appointment of a Health Care Agent) and a Living Will (now called an Advance Care Plan). (See Financial & Legal Issues Chapter.)

■ If you are caring for an elderly loved one, consider using as the primary care provider a doctor who is board certified in geriatrics.

If your loved one is able to actively participate in the health care process, your role may be more of a partner and support person in planning and preparing for encounters with healthcare professionals. You may also need to assume the role of an advocate to help him/her negotiate the health care system.

Medical Appointments

1. <u>Planning Ahead</u> is an important and essential part of getting the most from a medical appointment.

    ■ Try to schedule the appointment for your loved one's best time of day. You might also ask office staff what time of day or day of the week the office is least crowded.

    ■ If you have a number of concerns to discuss which may require more time than allotted for a typical appointment, let the office staff know in advance that you may need some additional time with the doctor.

- If the patient is memory-impaired and/or likely to be resistant or anxious about going to the doctor, wait until the day of the visit to inform them of the appointment and be positive and matter-of-fact.

- You may want to bring something for the patient to eat and drink, as well as an enjoyable activity, to help pass the time in the waiting room.

- Propose that a family member or friend go along to the appointment. In addition to providing moral support, another person may help to relay significant information to the healthcare provider or ask an important question that might otherwise be forgotten. If test results or other detailed or upsetting information may be given, another set of ears is helpful in remembering and understanding what has been told.

- Make a health care file which includes the patient's medical history and diagnoses, medications, allergies, emergency contacts, names and numbers of healthcare providers, health insurance information, and copies of advance directives, living wills, and/or durable power of attorney for healthcare. These are needed by hospitals upon admission and by specialists to whom the senior may be referred.

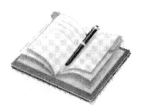

2. <u>Being Prepared</u> is the most effective approach to getting what you want from an appointment with a doctor or other health care professional. It also gives the medical staff the information necessary to make good healthcare decisions without the distraction of unnecessary or irrelevant details.

    ■ Write down what you want to discuss with the doctor or other health professional. Put your concerns in order of priority, so you will be sure to talk about the most important ones, even if you don't have time for all of them.

    ■ Make a list of any important changes and/or new symptoms since the last appointment, including any major changes or stressors in the patient's life, such as the death of a family member or a new living situation.

    ■ Briefly summarize general health information, including weight (loss or gain), appetite (increase or decrease), sleep patterns, restlessness or lethargy, and mood (depressed, withdrawn, anxious, upbeat).

    ■ Take with you, either all of the medications the patient is currently on, or a list of the medications, dosages, and frequencies. Include vitamins, over the counter medications, nutritional supplements, and herbal medicines.

    ■ Arrive early enough to fill out the office paperwork before the scheduled appointment time.

3.   <u>Taking Charge</u> of the appointment establishes your role as a vital member of the health care team. Identify yourself and the patient if needed, make eye contact, and let the medical staff person (nurse, doctor, physician's assistant, physical therapist, etc.) know that you are prepared to provide whatever information is needed, particularly if the patient is unable or unlikely to do so.

■   Be honest and factual in answering questions. Telling a doctor what you think he/she wants to hear will not help you or the patient obtain good medical care. If you need to share information that might be upsetting to the patient, ask ahead of time to speak to the doctor privately or provide that information prior to the appointment.

■   Stick to the point by focusing on the information you need to share and the concerns you want to address. Be brief but specific and descriptive.

■   Ask questions: this is a key to getting what you want from the visit. Ask for clarification, for more information, or about treatment options. Make notes for later reference or use a tape recorder (with the doctor's permission).

■   Repeating back to the doctor what you have heard is a good way to insure that you and the doctor are "on the same page."

■   Share your point of view. What the doctor or other health professional suggests as a plan of care may not be what works best for you as the caregiver. State your concerns and ask about other options.

- Whenever possible, have the doctor or the office staff provide written advice and instructions and/or refer to additional sources of information. If you are expecting test results, ask how and when you can expect to have the results relayed to you.

- Make a contingency plan. Ask the doctor what to expect and what to do if there is a problem, particularly outside of office hours. It is better to plan now than to try to figure it out when you are frantic at 3 a.m.

- Talk to other members of the health care team in addition to the doctor. Doctors may not be able to answer every question. For example, pharmacists are often the best source of information about possible drug side effects and drug interactions.

> You have an important role in helping your loved one follow through with the plan of care the doctor has recommended.

- Insure that medications and treatments are being given as prescribed – note dosage and frequency and monitor for potential side effects.

- Notify the doctor if the medication or treatment is not effective within the expected time frame or if there are side effects that concern you.

- Update the health care file following each doctor's visit to reflect any changes in the plan of care, new or discontinued medications, etc.

- Do your own research so that you and your loved one are informed and effective advocates. Bookstores, libraries, specific disease-related organizations (such as American Cancer Society or Alzheimer's Association), and the Internet offer a wealth of educational materials.

Hospitalization

From time of admission to discharge, your loved one's condition and care needs are being reviewed to make sure that the hospital is the only location of care that the treatment can be safely administered. As soon as care can be provided at another level, such as a skilled nursing home or at home, there will be discussion about discharging your family member from the hospital.

REMEMBER:

- The hospital staff should provide education prior to discharge regarding the needs of the patient who is returning home. Education may be provided by the nurse, the rehab therapist, the certified diabetes educator, the respiratory therapist, and/or others as appropriate. Ask for further education if you do not think you understand the instructions for care after discharge.

- Some seniors get disoriented in the hospital. This may also be true if the senior is going from the hospital to a new facility or a relative's home.

- Every hospital is required to have someone identified to help you with planning for care after discharge. This person may be a nurse case manager or a social worker. The "discharge planner" is available to help you review your options for care and to help you with arranging for any special needs of your loved one such as home medical equipment or home health care. If you need assistance with planning, ask for the "discharge planner" or nurse case manager or social worker.

■ If you think your family member is being discharged too soon, Medicare has a procedure to address this issue.

■ Every hospital has a process for examining ethical issues. Often this is an ethics committee. Patients and/or their families have a right to access this committee or process. You could ask for an ethics consult if there is a dilemma or disagreement about the course of treatment. You could request this if you need help with serious health care decisions that often have to be made at the end of life.

Home Health Care

To get home health through Medicare, an individual has to be "homebound" and require either skilled nursing or rehab services. A physician has to order services. When you are getting home health services, a primary case manager should be available to talk with you, with your elder's permission. Also, you can request that the physician order a social work visit if you need help with long-term care planning and decision making.

Nursing Facility / Assisted Living Facility

As a family member your caregiving does not end with nursing home placement or placement in an assisted living facility. As a caregiver and family member, you are partners with the facility in providing care to your elder. Helping the staff to know and understand your family member can enhance the quality of care received.

■ Write down information about your elder's care that will help the staff. If your elder has difficulty communicating preferences and needs, write these down in a notebook that can be shared with the staff. This is particularly helpful if your family member has multiple caregivers.

■ Develop positive relationships with the direct caregiver staff. Express appreciation to them when they do a good job.

■ Each nursing facility has regularly scheduled team meetings to review your elder's "care plan." Your elder and you as a family member should be invited to participate in this meeting. This is an opportunity for you to assist the team in the care of your elder. Assisted Living Facilities may not have regularly scheduled care plan meetings. However, you can request a meeting with key staff to discuss your loved one's needs.

■ If you have problems that you are not able to resolve by talking with direct care staff, supervisory staff, and/or administrative staff at the nursing home, you may contact your nursing home ombudsman for assistance.

Hospice

Hospice is a program for persons with life-threatening illness when the life expectancy is six months or less. Persons can be in hospice longer than six months if there is a continuing decline and if the hospice determines that continued eligibility is met. Hospice care is physician-directed and provided by a multi-disciplinary team. The focus is on symptom management and not on cure of the disease. Medicare has a special insurance benefit for hospice.

If your family member is in hospice, your needs as family caregiver are important to the hospice team. Not only does hospice attend to the multi-dimensional needs of the patient (physical, emotional, social,

> " ... your needs as family caregivers are important to the hospice team "

spiritual), but they also address the needs of the caregiving family. Open communication about your needs and concerns will assist the hospice team in caring for you and your older relative. Hospice will remain in contact with you after the death of your relative and will offer bereavement services as well.

See chapter on **End of Life Care for more information about Hospice.

Managing Medications

The average senior citizen takes 4.5 prescription and 2 over-the-counter medications daily. Managing multiple medications can at times be a difficult task. Some helpful hints to effectively manage medications for the senior:

- **Bring all medications (both prescribed and over-the-counter) to all doctor's visits.** You can also bring a list of all medications taken. It is important that your healthcare provider knows of all medications that the senior is taking.

- **Check first.** Never give an over-the-counter medication (including herbs and dietary supplements) without first checking with the patient's healthcare professional. Some of these medications may interact with other medications and could potentially cause harmful effects.

- **Compliance products.** Use a medication compliance product such as pillboxes, pill timers, or specialized pill packages. Talk with your pharmacist about this.

- **Schedule.** Ask the healthcare provider to write a schedule of when medications should be taken throughout the day and whether they should be taken with food or on an empty stomach.

- **Difficulty swallowing.** If the senior has difficulty swallowing medications, talk with the healthcare professional about an alternative form of the medication. Never crush medications without first talking to a healthcare professional.

- **Side effects.** If you suspect that a medication may be causing adverse effects in the senior, contact the healthcare provider before stopping this medication. Be observant for any changes that may occur when the senior first starts taking a medication.

- **Talk with your pharmacist.** Consult your pharmacist if you have any questions about your loved one's medications. It is especially important to ask what food or drink may interact with the senior's medications. Pharmacists' extensive knowledge about medications can be of great benefit to you.

- **Vision problems.** If the senior has difficulty reading pill bottles, it might be helpful to color-code pill bottles. For example, the senior may know to take one pill from the yellow bottle two times a day.

■ **Take all medications as prescribed.** It is important not to skip doses or double up if a dose is missed, as this could potentially cause adverse effects.

■ **Do not share medications with others.** Medications can behave differently in seniors than they do in younger adults.

■ **Use the same pharmacy for all medications.** It is important that your pharmacy has a complete record of medications to keep up with changes in dosages of medications and to be sure no interacting medications have been prescribed by different healthcare providers.

Over the Counter Medications

Many seniors take over the counter (OTC) medications. It is <u>very important</u> to notify your health care provider of any OTC medications taken, as some may interfere with prescribed medications or with different health problems. Listed below are common OTC medications with tips about their potential side effects and limitations in elderly individuals. If you or your loved one has any concern about medications, it is best to consult your pharmacist or health care provider to discuss these concerns.

PAIN RELIEVERS

■ **Acetaminophen** (Tylenol)
Elderly individuals should take no more than four grams (4000 mg) of Tylenol a day.

■ **Aspirin and NSAIDs**

The most frequent side effect of aspirin and NSAIDs (nonsteroidal anti-inflammatories) is gastrointestinal (GI) upset. Examples of over the counter NSAIDs are ibuprofen (Motrin or Advil) and naproxen (Naprosyn). Sometimes the prolonged use of NSAIDs can cause GI bleeding, more commonly in the elderly. This can also occur when NSAIDs are taken in high dosages or in those who have more than one alcoholic beverage per week while taking NSAIDs. These medications need to be used sparingly by those with kidney problems as well as those with high blood pressure.

■ **Antihistamines**

Antihistamines are medications that are used to treat allergy symptoms such as itching, nasal irritation, sneezing, and mucus production. They are also used at night to help treat insomnia. Three common OTC antihistamines are:

<u>Brompheniramine</u>: medicine in Dimetapp Allergy

<u>Diphenhydramine</u>: medicine in Benadryl and Tylenol PM

<u>Chlorpheniramine</u>: medicine in Chlor-Trimeton Allergy

Antihistamines can cause sedation or drowsiness and therefore can significantly impair a person's ability to drive and increase an individual's risk of falling. These medications can also cause urinary retention (lack of an ability to urinate), constipation, increased intraocular pressure (pressure inside of the eye), confusion, disorientation, and agitation. The combination of alcohol and antihistamines can cause increased drowsiness.

> These OTC antihistamines should be avoided
> or used as little as possible in the elderly.

▣ Decongestants

Pseudoephedrine: medicine in Sudafed

Phenylephrine: medicine in Sudafed PE

Decongestants are similar to adrenaline, and they cause blood vessels to constrict and therefore increase blood pressure or raise blood sugar levels. Pseudoephedrine can also cause nervousness and heart palpitations. It interacts with many prescription medications, including beta-blockers, antidepressants, and insulin. Elderly individuals who have high blood pressure, glaucoma, or diabetes should <u>never take an OTC decongestant without first checking with their healthcare provider</u>. Individuals taking certain types of antidepressant medications or medications for a seizure disorder should also avoid taking OTC decongestants.

▣ Cough medicines

Cough medicines are grouped into two categories: expectorants and antitussives. Expectorants thin the mucus, making it easier to clear it from the airway. Guaifenesin, one of the medicines in Robitussin, is an expectorant. Antitussives block the cough reflex. Dextromethorphan is an antitussive and is the product found in Drixoral, Delsym, Pertussin CS, and Robitussin. Dextromethorphan may cause confusion, agitation, nervousness, or irritability. Patients using a certain type of antidepressants (MAOI inhibitors) should not use dextromethorphan products.

Risk Factors for Medication Misuse

The biggest risk factor for seniors and medication misuse is from misuses such as:

- Taking extra doses

- Missing doses

- Not following instructions

- Using drugs that have expired

- Not knowing about side effects

- Sharing or borrowing drugs

- Taking the wrong drugs

- Mixing medications or drinking alcohol while taking medications

- Going to multiple physicians to get more of the same drug or multiple physicians prescribing multiple drugs

- Instructions and package inserts written in small print or confusing language

- Failure to tell the doctor about over-the-counter medications, megadose vitamins, or herbals

- Missing instructions as a result of hearing, vision, or memory problems.

(Adapted from *Substance Abuse & Mental Health Services Administration*)

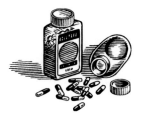

Mental
and
Emotional Health

Do you ever worry about your elder's mental health? Or wonder if his/her forgetfulness, moodiness, and loss of appetite are normal parts of aging? Are you concerned about a growing dependence on alcohol or drugs to deal with stressful events? It can be challenging to determine whether a noticeable change in disposition is due to external circumstances (e.g., death of a loved one, retirement) or internal health issues (e.g., chronic illness, medication side-effects, depression). Knowing what is a normal part of aging is important when deciding whether to seek assistance.

Moving, talking, and thinking a little more slowly are common as the body ages. As the nervous system becomes less efficient, older people often don't recall facts or respond to stimuli as quickly as they once did. However, persistent memory loss and confusion that interfere with daily life (e.g., wandering or getting lost in familiar surroundings, problems speaking, reading, and writing, and confusion with names and handling money) are NOT normal parts of aging. These symptoms may be signs of dementia, a medical condition that disrupts the way the brain works. Dementias may be either reversible (i.e., due to nutritional or thyroid imbalance) or irreversible (i.e., due to Alzheimer's disease, mini-strokes, or alcohol dependence). Only a thorough medical evaluation, which includes a mental status exam, can determine the cause and best treatment. It is estimated that 10 percent of adults ages 65 to74 and nearly half of those over 85 have Alzheimer's disease or a related dementia.

When you are concerned about your elder's mental health, it is important to seek information and assistance from a caring professional. You can call a local resource agency such as the Mental Health Association or the

Alzheimer's Association. You can also talk with your elder's physician, who may recommend an office visit or refer you to a geriatric psychiatrist for further testing. In more serious cases, an inpatient hospitalization may be the best course of action. The most important thing is to trust your intuition and seek assistance. By doing so, you will help your loved ones improve their quality of life and overall health and well-being.

Depression

Surveys have shown that a majority of older adults believe it is normal for people to get depressed as they grow older. However, depression is NOT a normal part of aging, but seniors are at an increased risk due to the likelihood of it occurring with other chronic health conditions (e.g., heart disease, stroke, Alzheimer's, cancer). Some medications (e.g., beta blockers) can cause depression as a side effect. Also, stressful life events (e.g., loss of a loved one or numerous friends, declining health, impaired mobility, and the loss of freedom associated with these declines) can trigger depression. Symptoms of depression include persistent sadness, change in eating habits with weight gain or loss, and change in sleeping habits. Given that primary care physicians accurately recognize less than one half of patients with depression and that seniors are more likely than any age group to try to handle depression themselves, it is important for you, as a caregiver, to communicate your concerns to your elder's physician. Left untreated, depression is a significant predictor of suicide among seniors, with older white males being particularly vulnerable. However, when recognized and addressed, clinical depression is a very treatable illness.

Contributing factors for depression in seniors are: loss of spouse or other family members, presence of chronic medical conditions, pain, loss of functional independence, frustration with memory loss, and difficulty adapting to changing circumstances.

> **Older adults typically do not complain of depression. What a caregiver may notice are sleeping problems (either can't sleep or sleeps much more than normal), agitation over small things, social withdrawal or isolation, clouding of mental awareness, or decline in the ability to take care of him/herself with daily activities.**
>
> **Seniors experiencing depression may be more willing to seek help from their primary care physician rather than a psychiatrist. There are many types of treatment for depression, and the physician can discuss these and make recommendations.**

Dementia

DEALING WITH THE DIAGNOSIS

Finding out that a loved one has Alzheimer's disease or another form of dementia can be stressful, frightening, and overwhelming. As you begin to take stock of the situation, here are some tips that may help:

- Ask the doctor any questions you have about dementia. Find out what treatments might work best to alleviate symptoms or address behavior problems.

■ Contact organizations such as the Alzheimer's Association and the Alzheimer's Disease Education and Referral (ADEAR) Center for more information about the disease, treatment options, and caregiving resources. Some community groups may offer classes to teach caregiving, problem-solving, and management skills.

■ Find a support group where you can share your feelings and concerns. Members of support groups often have helpful ideas or know of useful resources based on their own experiences. Online support groups make it possible for caregivers to receive support without having to leave home.

■ Study your day to see if you can develop a routine that makes things go more smoothly. If there are times of day when the person with dementia is less confused or more cooperative, plan your routine to make the most of those moments. Keep in mind that the way the person functions may change from day to day, so try to be flexible and adapt your routine as needed.

■ Consider using adult day care or respite services to ease the day-to-day demands of caregiving. These services allow you to have a break, while knowing that the person with dementia is being well cared for.

■ Begin to plan for the future. This may include getting financial and legal documents in order, investigating long-term care options, and determining what services are covered by health insurance and Medicare.

COMMUNICATION

Trying to communicate with a person who has dementia, particularly Alzheimer's disease, can be a challenge. Both understanding and being understood may be difficult.

- Choose simple words and short sentences and use a gentle, calm tone of voice.

- Avoid talking to the person with dementia as if they were a child or talking about the person as if they weren't there.

- Minimize distractions and noise—such as the television or radio—to help the person focus on what you are saying.

- Call the person by name, making sure you have his/her attention before speaking.

- Allow enough time for a response. Be careful not to interrupt.

- If the person with dementia is struggling to find a word or communicate a thought, gently try to provide the word he/she is looking for.

- Try to frame questions and instructions in a positive way.

- Be calm and quiet. Avoid using a loud tone of voice. Respect the person's personal space and don't get too close.

- Try to establish eye contact and call the person by name to get their attention. Remind the person who you are, if they doesn't seem to recognize you.

- If the person is confused, don't argue. Respond to the feelings you hear being communicated, and distract the person to a different topic if necessary.

- If the person doesn't recognize you, is unkind, or responds angrily, do not take it personally. He/she is reacting out of confusion.

DRIVING

Making the decision that a person with dementia is no longer safe to drive is difficult, and it needs to be communicated carefully and sensitively. Even though the person may be upset by the loss of independence, safety must be the priority.

- Look for clues that safe driving is no longer possible, including getting lost in familiar places, driving too fast or too slow, disregarding traffic signs, or getting angry or confused.

- Be sensitive to the person's feelings about losing the ability to drive, but be firm that he/she no longer do so. Be consistent—don't allow the person to drive on "good days" but forbid it on "bad days."

- Ask the doctor to help. The person may view the doctor as an "authority" and be willing to stop driving. The doctor also can contact the Department of Motor Vehicles and request that the person be reevaluated.

■ If necessary, take the car keys. If just having keys is important to the person, substitute a different set of keys.

■ If all else fails, disable the car or move it to a location where the person cannot see it or gain access to it.

BATHING

While some people with dementia don't mind bathing, for others it is a frightening, confusing experience.

■ Plan the bath or shower for the time of day when the person is most calm and agreeable. Be consistent. Try to develop a routine.

■ Respect the fact that bathing is scary and uncomfortable for some people with dementia. It is also something that previously was a very private activity. Be gentle, respectful, patient, and calm.

■ Tell the person what you are going to do, step by step, and allow him/her to do as much as possible.

■ Prepare in advance. Make sure you have everything you need ready and in the bathroom before beginning. Draw the bath ahead of time.

■ Be sensitive to the temperature. Warm up the room beforehand if necessary and keep extra towels and a robe nearby. Test the water temperature before beginning the bath or shower.

■ Minimize safety risks by using a handheld showerhead, shower bench, grab bars, and nonskid bath mats. Never leave the person alone in the bath or shower.

- Try a sponge bath. Bathing may not be necessary every day. A sponge bath can be effective between showers or baths.

DRESSING

For someone with dementia, getting dressed presents a series of challenges: choosing what to wear, getting some clothes off and other clothes on, and struggling with buttons and zippers. Minimizing the challenges may make a difference.

- Try to have the person get dressed at the same time each day, so he/she will come to expect it as part of the daily routine.

- Encourage the person to dress him/herself to whatever degree possible. Plan to allow extra time, so there is no pressure or rush.

- Allow the person to choose from a limited selection of outfits. If he/she has a favorite outfit, consider buying several identical sets.

- Arrange the clothes in the order they are to be put on to help the person move through the process.

- Provide clear, step-by-step instructions if the person needs prompting.

- Choose clothing that is comfortable, easy to get on and off, and easy to care for. Elastic waists and Velcro enclosures minimize struggles with buttons and zippers.

- Consider how slacks will fit with adult diapers if the senior is incontinent.

EATING

Eating can be a challenge. Some people with dementia want to eat all the time, while others have to be encouraged to maintain a good diet.

- View mealtimes as opportunities for social interaction. Try to be patient, to avoid rushing, and to be sensitive to confusion and anxiety.

- Aim for a quiet, calm, reassuring mealtime atmosphere by limiting noise and other distractions.

- Maintain familiar mealtime routines, but adapt to the person's changing needs.

- Give the person food choices, but limit the number of choices. Try to offer appealing foods that have familiar flavors, varied textures, and different colors.

- Serve small portions or several small meals throughout the day. Make healthy snacks, finger foods, and shakes available. In the earlier stages of dementia, be aware of the possibility of overeating.

- Choose dishes and eating tools that promote independence. If the person has trouble using utensils, use a bowl instead of a plate, or offer utensils with large or built-up handles. Use straws or cups with lids to make drinking easier.

- Encourage the person to drink plenty of fluids throughout the day to avoid dehydration.

- As the disease progresses, be aware of the increased risk of choking because of chewing and swallowing problems.

- Maintain routine dental checkups and daily oral health care to keep the mouth and teeth healthy.

ACTIVITIES

- What to do all day? Finding activities that the person with dementia can do, and is interested in, can be a challenge. Building on current skills generally works better than trying to teach something new.

- Don't expect too much. Simple activities often are best, especially when they use current abilities.

- Help the person get started on an activity. Break the activity down into small steps and praise the person for each step he/she completes.

- Watch for signs of agitation or frustration with an activity. Gently help or distract the person to something else.

- Incorporate activities the person seems to enjoy into your daily routine and try to do them at a similar time each day.

- Try to include the senior with dementia in the entire activity process. For instance, at mealtimes, encourage the person to help prepare the food, set the table, pull out the chairs, or put away the dishes. This can help maintain functional skills, enhance feelings of personal control, and make good use of time.

Take advantage of adult day services, which provide various activities for the person with dementia, as well as an opportunity for caregivers to gain temporary relief from caregiving. Transportation and meals often are provided.

Resources

- **Aging & Disability Resource Connection**   1-877-973-6467

  As part of the Area Agency on Aging & Disability, it offers information and some services or financial assistance.

- **Alzheimer's Association, Mid South Chapter**   1-800-272-3900

  Provides referral to local support groups and operates several programs to provide relief and assistance to families.

- **Mental Health Association of Middle Tennessee**   1-866-535-3825

  Offers caregiver training, information, and referrals.

Staying

at

Home

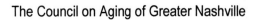

As a senior becomes more frail, either physically or mentally, the caregiver's concern with the practicality of keeping a loved one at home increases. The dilemma over whether or not to stay at home with support or move to a retirement community, assisted living facility, or nursing home becomes an issue. The thought of downsizing and moving to an unfamiliar new place can be daunting, as well as the fear of having less independence. Also, the impact of such a dramatic change in lifestyle can sometimes cause more harm than good. The following list of questions and knowledge of available resources may help your family in making a final decision. Long distance caregiving increases the dilemma, for the caregiver cannot "check in" as often.

Financial Considerations

Is a long-term care insurance policy in place? Does it cover in-home services? What is the waiting period? Is an evaluation of the senior required? If so, have you contacted the primary care doctor to assist in the insurance company's health evaluation? How many hours of care does it cover for hired caregivers? Does it cover special aids such as walkers or wheel chairs?

If long-term care insurance is not in place, have you tallied the daily costs of staying at home-- such as salaries and taxes for hired caregivers, utilities, home and yard maintenance and repairs, groceries, housekeeping, etc.?

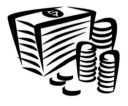

Socialization Considerations

As a senior loses mobility and can no longer drive, he/she can start to feel the effects of isolation and long lonely days. If a senior chooses to stay at home, the following questions should be addressed:

■ Is there an Adult Day Care facility, church group, or senior center nearby that can provide stimulating programs for socialization (lectures, bridge, games, volunteer opportunities, etc.) or fitness activities?

■ If there is a live-in family caregiver, is respite care available to provide several hours of personal time for the caregiver during the week? Caregiving agencies exist that provide respite services as well as 24-hour per day coverage for seniors and disabled individuals. Have a backup plan if the caregiver is out with sickness or a vacation. Some assisted living or nursing home facilities provide short term stays for just such situations.

■ Have friends, family members, neighbors, or the congregation (many churches have Stephen Ministers who are trained to visit homebound seniors) been encouraged to visit or to telephone (both to see if the senior needs anything and just to chat) on a regular basis?

■ Has the senior taken advantage of the resources available through the public library that can lessen loneliness or boredom, such as free videos, books on tape, and large print books that can be ordered over the phone? Is there someone who can tape favorite shows to be watched at later times?

■ If the senior is unable to read due to vision impairment or loss of ability to concentrate, is there someone who can read to him/her each day? The Library for the Blind has a free service for audio books. Check with your local public library.

■ Has he/she been encouraged to learn how to use the computer--a great way for keeping in touch with family and friends via e-mail, keeping current with the news, shopping, etc?

■ Is there a radio that can be set at a special channel for music or news?

■ Have a phone beside the bed.

■ Have an emergency plan in place for power outages.

Meal Considerations

Another concern for seniors living at home is whether they are receiving proper nutrition, as well as the safety issues involved with cooking. As both appetite and physical/mental capabilities diminish, it is important to be sure the following issues have been addressed:

■ If the elder is on medication, is there a failsafe method to ensure that daily meds are taken at the appropriate time with or without food (as prescribed) and that they are stored in a container clearly marked in large print for each day: a.m. and p.m.?

■ Is there a fire extinguisher in the kitchen (as well as other rooms) that the senior knows how to use and would be able to operate?

■ Is the senior still able to read the instructions on food packages and turn the knobs on oven and burners? If not, has there been instruction on use of microwave? (A caregiver can prepare meals on plates in advance to be reheated later.)

- Is a schedule in place so that he/she will eat breakfast, lunch, and dinner at regular hours?

- Is the senior aware of "Meals on Wheels" or "Mobile Meals," programs where volunteers deliver one hot meal five days a week to the home? Not only does it ensure one good meal; it also means that there will be someone "checking in" on a daily basis.

- Are fresh fruit and other easy-access foods kept available?

- Is there someone to check the refrigerator once a week to see what is needed from the grocery store and to check expiration dates on perishables?

Home Assessment for Mobility and Safety

When a senior chooses to remain at home, there are adaptations that will make living alone easier and safer and give more peace of mind to the senior, family, and caregivers. Insurance will sometimes pay for specific devices and/or modifications. Even small changes in the home can improve safety and enable seniors to remain there longer.

Too, exercise helps. Modest weight lifting and Tai-Chi, are known to improve balance and strength, while walking and gardening can keep one healthy and in good shape. However, falls are a continuing concern and risk.

Falls, though, are an issue. One in three seniors over 65 will fall each year. Only 10% of those who get help within 12 hours will be able to return to an independent home. The traditional (and a good) solution in personal emergency response systems (PERS or medical alarm systems) is a panic button worn as a pendant or bracelet that can be pressed to bring assistance. Still, data show that many older adults will not wear the button, let alone be able to use it in an emergency. But, advances in technology have progressed now to simple, mobile systems, which provide real-time, "intelligent," in-home monitoring, via customized sensors, which can monitor both user AND their home for signs that an emergency or problem might have occurred and then send instant alerts, within the house, and to those designated (i.e. family members, caregivers, neighbors, 911 etc.), who can provide the most appropriate help for the situation.

Checklist for Preventing Falls in the Home

	ALL ROOMS
	Use carpet with short dense pile.
	Apply double-sided carpet tape to rugs that can slip.
	Arrange furniture so you can walk easily around it.
	Make sure electrical and extension cords are not in your walking path.
	Make sure you can turn on lights without having to walk through dark areas.
	Use nightlights.
	Keep exits and hallways clear.
	Use stable chairs with armrests to help you get up.
	Provide bright, evenly distributed light.
	Use window shades that reduce glare.
	Make sure you can easily reach a light switch when you come into a room.
	Have more than one phone in the house.
	Make sure surfaces are safe and non-slip.
	Avoid scatter rugs or door mats that may be dangerous.
	Make sure changes in levels are obvious or marked in some way.

STAIRS	
	Put handrails on both sides of the steps.
	Make sure steps are even.
	Use non-skid contrasting tape, rubber stair treads, or coated skid resistant surface treatment on non-carpeted stairs. Apply tape to dry, clean surfaces at one-inch intervals. Use three long strips of tape on each step.
	Make sure electrical and extension cords are not in your walking path.
	Check carpeting to make sure it is firmly attached along stairs.
	Make repairs to worn or loose carpet promptly.
	Select a carpet pattern that doesn't hide the edge of steps, making you think steps have ended when they haven't.
	Don't place throw or scatter rugs at the top or bottom of stairways. All rugs should be secured firmly to the floor.
	Use good lighting (at least 60 watt bulbs) in the stairway. Install on/off switches at the top and bottom of stairs.
	Never leave books, purses, packages, or other objects on stairs.
	Watch out for a single step. People often trip when there is only one step.
	Avoid hurrying or not paying attention when on the stairs.
	Be especially careful when one carries large loads or wears shoes that are easy to slip in.

KITCHEN	
	Use sturdy stepstools – preferably with handrails.
	Throw out any stepstools that have broken parts.
	Clean spills immediately to avoid slipping.

BATHROOM
Use rubber bathmats or strips in bathtubs and showers.
Install at least two grab bars in the bath.
Clean up water from the floor.
Use raised toilet seats and/or handrails, securely fastened, if the person is at all unsteady.
Use a nightlight.

OUTSIDE
Install handrails along any flight of outdoor steps.
Spread sand on icy walkways.
Clean spills or slippery surfaces in garages immediately, before walking on them – especially oil or grease on cement floors.

WINDOWS AND DOORS
Make sure windows/doors are easy to open/close.
Make sure locks are sturdy/easy to operate.
Make sure doors are wide enough for a walker/wheelchair.
Check that door thresholds are not raised too high.
Create space to maneuver while opening/closing doors.
Create a view panel for the front door.
The view panel should be at a proper height for the resident.

MEDICATION
Store all medications out of the reach of children.
Secure all caps on medication bottles.
Store syringes behind a closed door, and do not talk about the fact that you have syringes in your home.
Never expose medication, in or out of bottles, to sunlight. (This precaution also applies to injectable medications, such as insulin).

	ELECTRICAL OUTLETS AND SWITCHES
	Outlets/switches should be easy to turn on and off.
	Outlets should be properly grounded to prevent electrical shock.
	Extension cords should be in good condition.
	Are they needed?
	Smoke detectors should be placed in all necessary areas.
	Know how the alarm system, if any, works.
	The telephone should be readily available for emergencies.
	The telephone should be equipped for hearing enhancement if necessary.
	The doorbell should be audible in every part of the house.
	Check heating pads for cracks prior to use.
	If your family member must use an electrical life-sustaining device, notify the power company so that power can be restored promptly during an emergency.

	OXYGEN
	Place "No Smoking" placards on all entrances to your home. These placards are provided by the oxygen company.
	Do not use more than 50 feet of tubing between the oxygen source and the patient.
	Do not place oxygen tanks within 1 ½ feet of windows/doors or other objects.
	Roll the tubing and carry it to avoid tripping and falling when walking.
	Do not have open flames, such as pilot lights of gas stoves or water heaters, within 12 feet of any oxygen equipment. (This warning applies to tubing, too).
	Place the telephone number of your electric company on or at every telephone. Call in the event of a power outage.

Disposal of Hazardous Materials

A. NEEDLES

- Never recap needles.

- Place needles and syringes inside a metal can with a lid.

- Store needles and syringes out of reach of children and out of sight of visitors.

- When the can is three-fourths full, place can (without lid) in oven for one hour at 350 degrees to melt syringes.

B. DRAINAGE WASTE

- Place all used dressings in a plastic bag and place it inside your household trash plastic bag.

- Wash hands thoroughly with soap and water before and after contact with waste.

- Disinfect soiled clothing by washing separately in hot water with bleach.

Additional In-Home Support

As a result of the emotional and physical stresses associated with long-term caregiving for an elder at home, there is often a time when outside support becomes necessary. In-home care, also called "personal support services," is defined as non-medical, personal support, custodial services. Service providers can offer anywhere from one to 24 hours of care, and no doctor's order is required. However, long-term care insurance, depending on the policy, may or may not cover these services.

Services include but are not limited to: transportation (to and from doctor's appointments and social activities), light housekeeping, meal preparation, medication reminders, bathing and grooming assistance, and companionship. Agencies that provide these services should be licensed with the state (a requirement in Tennessee).

Numerous agencies exist that provide trained helpers who range from nurses to sitters/professional caregivers. There are also service providers

> " Numerous agencies exist that provide trained helpers ... "

that can help with all other day-to-day management of the senior's life (i.e., bill pay services, management of petty cash, maintenance of home, shopping, etc.). Some of the best help can be found through word of mouth. The process of finding someone dependable and good, however, can be quite challenging. Below are a few tips to keep in mind while choosing an appropriate caregiver for your family:

- Research the reputation of each agency thoroughly. (A list of licensed agencies is included in the Council on Aging's Directory of Services for Seniors).

- Interview prospective employees before they meet with the senior. If they seem to meet with your requirements, be sure that the senior is involved in the hiring process. It is important that he/she feels comfortable with this new person in his/her daily life.

- Ask for references and follow through by calling them.

- Make sure a thorough criminal background check in all states of residence for the last ten years has been conducted on anyone coming into your home. Because background checks can differ, if you use an agency, always address specific issues. If you prefer to hire an independent contractor, you should contact a professional company specializing in this kind of business. Check "Employment Screening Companies" in the yellow pages. Also check the TN Department of Health Nurse Aide/Elder Abuse Registry at 1-800-778-4504.

- Check to see if the applicant is a smoker. If so, set guidelines for smoking areas and time allotment.

- Present a written list of expectations, as well as a contract stating salary, holiday pay (some request time and a half), withholding tax, etc.

- Before signing a contract, it is essential first to have a "trial run."

- Keep in mind that fewer faces, and consequently fewer changes and adjustments, are the ideal. Try to make a schedule that is consistent.

- Ask hired caregivers to wear a nametag with big print.

- Have the helper answer the phone by giving first the name of the resident followed by his/her own name. Always keep a notepad and pen handy to record messages even if the senior is not asleep. It is helpful for both the senior (who might suffer from short-term memory loss) and family members to know who has called. (When the senior is taking a nap, have the phone "turned down" or off in that room to ensure a good rest).

■ Ask if the agency conducts pre-employment or scheduled, random drug screens on employees.

Some Qualities to Look for in a Professional Caregiver

A. A PROFESSIONAL APPEARANCE

Appearance provides clues about a person's attitude and professionalism. One should be clean, well-groomed, and dressed appropriately for the job. Try to look beyond generational norms— blue hair does not mean a person is a bad caregiver! Don't be fooled by size: some large people move quickly and smoothly. By the same measure, a slight, slim person may be quite strong. The important factors are that one is well-trained and uses the proper equipment.

B. GOOD OBSERVATIONAL SKILLS

A good caregiver is observant and sensitive to changes in the senior's condition. In evaluating this, have the caregiver interact with the senior. Together you can judge whether the caregiver seems to have a "feel" for the person and the situation, as well as the skills to identify and deal with the senior's physical and emotional needs. Trust your instincts.

C. GOOD COMMUNICATION SKILLS

The ability to communicate with persons with perceptual problems may make caregivers seem rather odd at first! Accustomed to working with hearing-impaired or visually-impaired persons, they may speak more loudly and slowly than you are used to. Or they may ask questions not normally asked on an interview. However, good intuition can be much appreciated by someone who can't verbalize his/her needs. Note if they look the senior in the eye. Or use touch. Or give the senior time to respond.

D. QUIET SELF-CONFIDENCE

Arrogance and "an attitude" are not helpful; a sense of quiet self-confidence is. After all, part of the job is to give reassurance to you and your loved one. You need to feel you are both in good hands.

E. AN OPEN MIND

Good caregivers must be tolerant and accepting of ideas and beliefs that may not be their own. Care receivers are often different from their caregivers in age, gender, ethnicity, and beliefs. They often take out feelings of frustration, anger, or other strong emotion, blurting out insults or even physically striking out at the caregiver. An experienced caregiver will not take this behavior personally but will try to assess the issue or circumstances and respond appropriately.

F. A SENSE OF HUMOR AND CREATIVITY

For caregivers, who often face many challenges with clients who are dealing with a variety of issues, an even temperament and a sense of humor can avert many potential crises. Creative problem-solving in helping the senior to maintain a sense of dignity, respect, and even autonomy is an important quality for delivering care in a professional and nurturing manner.

Begin with a two-week trial with an evaluation by all parties midway through. Comfort with the caregiver is important, but competence is essential!

Home Health Care

In the formal definition of home health care, the basic components are nursing care, social work, therapies (speech therapy, physical therapy, occupational therapy), and limited health aide services. These are ordered by a physician and are short-term.

Most home health care is reimbursed through the Medicare and Medicaid systems. Generally, these two programs focus on illness care and have strict eligibility criteria. Home health covers skilled care services on an intermittent basis that are ordered by the physician to assist patients 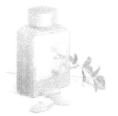 and families through a bout of illness. The patient must be home-bound and require medically necessary care. Home health agencies are regulated through state licensure and Medicare/Medicaid certification.

For individuals who require in-home care but are not eligible for Medicare or Medicaid, there are benefits available through commercial insurance, private pay, long-term care insurance and special waiver programs managed through state, local, and other federal funding. In addition to intermittent care, some in-home agencies can offer extended private-duty care in the home that may in some instances be covered by the patient's insurance program. Again, it is important to determine that the agency providing care meets licensure and credentialing standards, which offer consumer protection.

Medication Management

When a senior is unable to manage medications independently and the family or professional caregiver becomes responsible, there are several systems that can be put in place. New technology is available that reminds the senior at the appropriate time to take a pre-loaded dose of his/her medication. Some systems also have the capability of reminding the senior of various other important health-related items (i.e., blood sugar checks, food thirty minutes before medications, etc.).

These systems assist in continuity of the medication regimen, which in turn allows the senior to remain independent longer. Nurses and care managers can help in locating and managing these systems.

Mismanagement of medications is the most common reason for hospital admissions for seniors.

Avoiding Scams

Everyone, but especially seniors living alone, should be alert to the ways scam artists operate. Seniors should be given the following advice:

- Never respond to phone solicitations for products or winning sweepstake numbers.

- Key words that should arouse suspicion: cash only, get rich quick, something for nothing, contests, haste, today only.

- Never release personal information to anyone who contacts you.

- Do not give your credit card or Social Security information over the phone UNLESS YOU HAVE INITIATED THE CALL.

- Beware of someone contacting you with information about lost relatives.

- When approached for a donation, find out what charity or business is involved. If you have not heard of this charity, ask for written information. They will send it if they are a legitimate organization. If not, it is most likely a scam.

- Check out any contractor coming to do work on your home. Ask for the contractor's state license number. Call the TN Board of Licensing Contractors at (615) 741-8307 or the TN Home Improvement Board at (615) 741-5630 to confirm that the contractor has an active license and has posted the required bond.

- Check the standing of the business or service with the Better Business Bureau.

- Beware of unsolicited door-to-door sales; under the law, you may cancel a door-to-door sale within three business days of the sale by notifying the seller in writing.

Financial Exploitation

Older consumers lose millions of dollars each year because of financial exploitation. This may be the result of an unknown con artist's scam or financial abuse by someone the victim knows well. Financial exploitation is defined as the "illegal or improper use of an adult's resources or property." The National Center for Elder Abuse in Washington, D. C. indicates that financial exploitation accounts for about 12 percent of all reported elder abuse cases. This may be only a portion of actual cases, however, because victims often are too ashamed or embarrassed to report this type of crime. Everyone wants to help one's family and friends, and it may be hard, for example, to refuse a favorite grandchild's request to co-sign a car loan. However, keep in mind that the co-signer will be liable for the loan if the family member is unable to pay.

If you think someone is being swindled by a person who tries to gain trust with a friendly and honest face or pleasant authoritative voice, ask these questions:

- Has someone told you that you need home repairs and demanded an immediate cash payment? Has anyone offered to accompany you to the bank for a quick withdrawal? Has anyone asked you to withdraw your money for any reason?

- Has a stranger asked you to put up "good faith" money so you can share in unexpectedly found valuables or cash?

- Has a stranger offered to "bless your money," remove a curse from it, or perform a ritual that will cause it to increase in value?

- Have you received a telephone call or visit from an alleged employee of a regulatory agency or bank examiner who claims to need your help in trapping a teller who may have been withdrawing money from your account?

PROTECTIONS FROM FINANCIAL EXPLOITATION:

- Consider having utility, phone, newspaper and other regular bills automatically paid by electronic transfer from checking or savings accounts.

- Consider direct deposit for benefit, pension or Social Security checks to reduce the opportunity for theft.

- Stay in regular contact with a number of friends and family members. Be watchful of a caregiver that tries to isolate the senior.

- Talk with the bank. Financial institutions are in a unique position to have early knowledge of on-going financial exploitation of older consumers. However, they will not give information to anyone who is not an owner of the account.

- Remember oral promises are not binding, especially if a written contract exists and does not agree with the oral promise.

- Don't leave a hidden key outside.

Resources

- *Clinical Pathways for the Multidisciplinary Home Care Team*
  – Barbara Stover Gingerich and Deborah Anne Ondeck

- *Home Safe Home, How to Prevent Falls in the Home* and *How Well Does Your Home Meet Your Needs*
  -- AARP: The Coalition for Consumer Health and Safety

The Tennessee Regulatory Authority has several programs to help those with hearing or vision problems access telephone services. Contact this department at 1-800-342-8359.

Transportation

We all want to maintain our independence by driving as long as possible. The fear of losing independence--and thus possibly having to move from home--keeps many seniors driving when it is no longer safe to do so.

Some signs that driving has become a problem:

- Feeling more nervous while driving.

- More traffic tickets or warnings in the last year.

- More dents or scratches on the car or on curbs, garage walls, or doors, etc.

- Trouble consistently staying in a single lane of traffic.

- Friends not wanting to ride with you.

- Trouble seeing or following road signs and pavement markings.

- Difficulty in concentrating while driving.

- Medications that may be affecting your ability to concentrate or drive safely.

- Medical conditions that may affect your driving ability.

- Response time to unexpected situations is slower than it used to be.

- Trouble moving your foot from the gas to the brake pedal.

- Getting lost more often.

- Difficulty in judging gaps in traffic at intersections and on entrance/exit ramps.

■ More frequent "close calls."

■ Other drivers honking at you more often.

■ Trouble seeing the sides of the road when you are looking ahead(cars/people "coming out of nowhere").

Those concerned about a senior's mental or physical ability to continue driving can seek help in several ways:

■ **AARP Driver Safety Program**   1-888-227-7669

This course (two four-hour sessions) is designed by AARP to alert seniors to normal age-related changes that affect driving capabilities. The course is also intended to help drivers improve their skills. Tennessee requires insurance companies to discount the cost of collision coverage for those seniors who successfully complete the course. There is a small fee for the classes. AARP also offers an online course (http://www.aarp.org/drive/online) that can be completed at one's own pace.

■ **Family doctor or ophthalmologist can intervene**

Call before an appointment and ask that the senior be evaluated regarding the ability to drive. The doctor can be the deliverer of the unwelcome news.

■ **Disable the car for dementia patients**

1. Disconnect the negative battery cable (usually black).
2. File key so that it does not start the car.

▪ Driver Evaluation

These programs are designed to evaluate the driving abilities of the disabled or elderly, including physical, psychological, perceptual, and cognitive status. Necessary adaptive driving equipment and training may be recommended.

On the Road Evaluations   615-294-3825

943 Woodland St., Nashville, TN 37206

Pi Beta Phi Rehab Institute   615-936-5040
Vanderbilt Bill Wilkerson Center

1215 21st Ave. S., Nashville, TN 37232

Many seniors self-limit their driving. They may no longer drive at night or in rainy weather. They may no longer drive to new places or to locations where interstate highway driving is necessary. They may go to only a few familiar places near their home such as church, grocery, or drugstore.

More action may be called for if the senior fails to recognize his/her declining ability. If someone diagnosed with dementia or early stage Alzheimer's disease continues to drive, there could be legal liability.

As you talk with the senior, emphasize that you don't want them to get hurt or hurt someone else. Help find other means of transportation. There may be church members in the neighborhood who would be glad to pick up your senior for services. There are also personal support service agencies that provide transportation for a fee. Many transportation programs are small and only serve certain neighborhoods or on certain days.

There may be a minimum of hours, so work to consolidate trips and appointments. A good birthday or holiday gift is to pay for a certain number of trips with one of these services.

Travel training is a new service in some communities. The local transit system will instruct new riders on using the bus system, will accompany them on several trips, and then give a free pass for a period of time.

Alternatives to Driving

PRIVATE CAR

- Family

- Friends

- Congregational groups

- Taxi

- Home care related services

For a listing of personal support agencies offering home care services, see the Council on Aging's *Directory of Services for Seniors* in the chapter 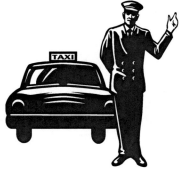 entitled "In-Home Services." Many options are listed, both private and non-profit.

SEMI-PRIVATE

■ Special agencies (e.g., the American Cancer Society) offer rides to medical appointments in many locations.

■ Assisted Living facilities generally provide transportation for their residents.

■ All Middle Tennessee counties provide ambulance service for non-life-threatening needs.

PUBLIC TRANSIT SYSTEMS

■ Metro Transit Authority, Customer Service   615-862-5950
A senior discount is available with an MTA Golden Age or Medicare card.

■ MTA Accessride   615-880-3970
Transportation for those who cannot use the regular bus service. Service is by reservation at least 24 hours in advance. The individual must be medically certified.

■ C.T.S. Bus Information   931-553-2429
Serving Clarksville and Fort Campbell, the system offers special senior fares.

■ Para-Transit LIFT Service   931-553-2470
Curb to curb service for disabled citizens in Clarksville.

■ Franklin Transit Authority   615-790-4005
Seniors can ride at a discounted cost.

- Transit on Demand (TODD) of Franklin Transit Authority   615-628-3344

- Murfreesboro Public Transportation (Rover)   615-494-1233

- Mid-Cumberland Human Resource Agency

  Offers curb-to-curb, accessible shared-ride transportation within outlying counties and into Davidson County.

Cheatham County	615-792-7242
Dickson County	615-446-4943
Houston County	931-289-4118
Humphreys County	931-296-2871
Montgomery County	931-647-4602
Robertson County	615-384-9335
Rutherford County	615-890-2677
Stewart County	931-232-6416
Sumner County	615-452-7433
Trousdale County	615-374-3311
Williamson County	615-790-5791
Wilson County	615-444-7433

Be aware of the pain of the loss of independence, loneliness, and grief when one is no longer able to drive.

Resources

- *We Need to Talk, Family Conversations with Older Drivers*
  -- AARP

Nutrition
for
Older Adults

The aging process progresses at different rates among individuals because of overall health, lifestyle, and genetic tendencies. However, nutritional status remains consistently important. Good nutrition throughout life is vital because it:

- Improves quality of life

- Supports immune function

- Helps the body resist infection

- Encourages faster healing from surgery or other wounds

- Maintains strong bones and muscle

- Increases energy level

- Contributes to improved outcomes from medical treatments

- May shorten the length of hospitalizations

Eating Right

Guidelines for good nutrition that include eating a variety of foods each day have been established by experts. In spite of special diet requirements ordered by physicians, most older adults should be able to include the following foods:

- **6 - 8** eight-ounce servings of water or other non-alcoholic liquids each day to help prevent dehydration and constipation. Fruit juice, milk, tea, or coffee all count towards this goal. The elderly have a decreased thirst response, so they might not always state they are thirsty when they actually need to drink.

- **6 or more** servings of bread, fortified or enriched cereal, rice or pasta. Choosing nutrient-rich whole grains such as brown rice, whole-wheat pastas, and bran cereals add fiber and improve the quality of the diet.

- **5 or more** servings of fruits or vegetables. Brightly colored foods (dark green, yellow, orange, or red) are typically higher in nutrients and good sources of fiber.

- **2 or more** servings (about 3-4 ounces each) of lean meat, poultry, fish, eggs, peanut butter, or dried beans. These foods are necessary for protein.

- **3 or more** servings of dairy products. These foods add protein to the diet and provide calcium and vitamin D to help maintain bone health

The amounts of food may vary depending on calorie and protein needs, and occasional modifications may need to be made based on medical conditions, special dietary restrictions, and physician recommendations.

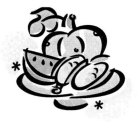

Senior citizens should consume 1500-2400 mg of sodium daily, but frequently older adults need to restrict sodium/salt intake because of a medical condition. If so, the following suggestions may be helpful:

■ Select fresh, frozen, or unsalted canned vegetables.

■ Use fresh, frozen, or canned fruits. They are naturally low in sodium.

■ Eat fresh (rather than processed) meats such as poultry, beef, fish, and pork. Check the labels of canned and frozen fish for added salt.

■ Limit high sodium items such as canned soups, bacon, sausage, ham, luncheon meats, salted snack items, frozen meals, and many fast food and restaurant meals.

■ Avoid high sodium seasonings (salt, seasoning salt, lemon pepper, bouillon, soy sauce, meat tenderizer). Instead, season with herbs, low sodium seasonings, fresh onion, and fresh garlic.

■ Low sodium salt substitutes ("Nu-Salt" and "No Sal") are high in potassium. Be sure to ask the health care provider if it is advisable to use these products.

Barriers to Good Nutrition

In spite of having knowledge of good nutrition and access to adequate food, many older adults have difficulty maintaining an acceptable intake. Risk factors for poor appetite, weight loss, and malnutrition may include:

- Impaired vision

- Decreased functional status

- Side-effects from medications that contribute to poor appetite

- Dementia

- Depression and anxiety

- Poorly fitting dentures, missing teeth, mouth sores

- Alcohol abuse

- Overall medical condition

- Swallowing problems -- coughing, choking, or throat clearing after eating or drinking

- Limited income

- Lack of social/family support

- Constipation -- can cause decreased appetite and nausea

Usually the first (and most important) sign of inadequate intake is unintentional weight loss. Checking weight two to four times each month will help monitor weight status.

POSSIBLE RECOMMENDATIONS:

- Manage/treat depression.

- Obtain an evaluation by a speech pathologist to assess swallowing function if problems are suspected (physician referral needed).

- Obtain an evaluation by a physical and/or occupational therapist if declining function is noted (physician referral needed) and adaptive equipment is needed.

- Obtain a nutritional evaluation by a registered dietitian. (Physician referral may be needed, depending on insurance.)

- Obtain a dental evaluation for possible dentures or denture modifications.

- Provide feeding assistance, as indicated.

- Evaluate possible medication-related causes of poor appetite (pharmacist and physician).

- Maintain regular bowel function.

- Increase activity level, if possible. This can build muscle, improve strength, and increase appetite.

- Liberalize modified diets. <u>Sometimes having an overly-restrictive diet can cause decreased intake.</u>

- Pay attention to food preferences.

- Make mealtimes social events. Include family members and eat together when possible.

- Provide softer foods if the older family member has chewing or swallowing problems. Use gravies and sauces to moisten drier foods. Older adults with advanced dementia may need foods that they can eat with their fingers instead of using eating utensils.

- Provide extra snacks between meals if the older adult can eat only small portions at regular mealtimes.

- Add nutritional supplements or high calorie/high protein foods to improve overall intake.

- Have larger meals earlier in the day. Older adults usually eat better at breakfast and lunch, but they want a lighter evening meal.

- Consider a multivitamin if intake is not adequate, especially if few vegetables or fruits are eaten.

- Don't forget the importance of adequate fluid intake.

Nutritional Issues Experienced by Older Adults

POOR APPETITE

When older adults experience a decrease in the frequency and quantity of food intake, poor appetite may be a concern. Poor appetite can be caused by difficulty swallowing, changed sense of taste or smell, depression, or pain.

- **Indications of Poor Appetite:** Difficulty swallowing, weight loss, lack of interest in food.

- **Suggestions**: Provide small, frequent meals of favorite foods. Try foods high in calories that are easy to eat (e.g., pudding, ice cream, or milk shakes). Encourage eating with friends and family. Provide beverages between meals instead of with meals since liquids may cause an early feeling of fullness.

CONSTIPATION

Constipation can cause a great deal of discomfort for older adults. Constipation may be influenced by age-related changes in the digestive tract, a lack of activity, general weakness, pain medication, and decreased fluid intake.

- **Indication of Constipation:** Stomach ache or cramps, no regular bowel movement within the past three days, excessive gas, or feelings of discomfort.

- **Suggestions:** Increase the amount of high-fiber foods (e.g., whole grain breads, fresh raw fruits and vegetables, and prune juice. Avoid foods and beverages that cause gas (e.g., cabbage, broccoli, and carbonated drinks). Increase fluid intake. Warm fluids in the morning, for example, may be helpful.

DEHYDRATION

Proper fluid intake is very important for older adults. Decreases in hydration can contribute to confusion and unsteadiness. As we age, most people begin to lose the sensation of thirst. Therefore, have the senior drink at regular intervals throughout the day, regardless of whether he or she feels thirsty. Experts recommend that all adults (unless instructed by a doctor to limit intake of fluids) drink at least eight glasses of fluid, 8 ounces each, every day.

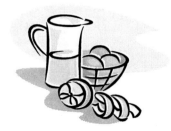

■ **Indication of dehydration:** Dizziness, weakness, inability to swallow dry food, dry skin, weight loss, little or no urine, and fatigue.

■ **Suggestions:** Use ice chips for relief of dry mouth. Increase intake of fluids. Increase intake of foods that contain fluids (e.g., fruits and soups). Keep fluids near the individual at all times for easy access.

SWALLOWING PROBLEMS (DYSPHAGIA)

Chewing and swallowing may be difficult for older adults with oral problems such as mouth sores, cavities, poorly fitting dentures, or untreated gum disease. This is a serious problem that can interfere with proper food intake and may put a senior at risk for medical complications related to aspiration of food or liquids into his or her lungs. If you notice changes in your loved one's ability to chew or swallow food, notify the doctor right away.

■ **Indications of swallowing problems:** Gagging, coughing, or regurgitation of food, loss of weight, and food building up in the mouth.

■ **Suggestions:** Provide soft, moist foods. Mash or blenderize foods (e.g., meats, cereals, fresh fruits). Provide liquids that have some consistency (e.g., blenderized fruits or milk shakes) because they are easier to swallow than clear liquids. Give small bites (1 teaspoon at a time). Make sure that the senior is in an upright position when eating and drinking.

When swallowing problems arise, health professional may suggest a *mechanical soft diet*. The mechanical soft diet is made up of regular table foods that are soft, moist, and easy to chew and swallow. This diet decreases the amount of chewing that a person must do while eating; it also allows him or her to have better control over foods in the mouth. It has the name "mechanical" because household tools and machines, like a blender, meat grinder, or knife, are used to make food easier to chew or swallow. The level of difficulty in swallowing should determine the consistency of the food.

DYSPHAGIA DIET: 5 LEVELS FOR DIFFICULTY IN SWALLOWING

LEVEL 1:	Pureed Foods (smooth, mashed potato-like consistency)
LEVEL 2:	Minced Foods (very small flecks of food, 1/8 inch, similar to size of sesame seed)
LEVEL 3:	Ground Foods (ground/diced into 1/4 inch pieces, similar to size of rice)
LEVEL 4:	Chopped Foods (cut into ½ inch pieces, similar to size of uncooked elbow macaroni)
LEVEL 5:	Modified Regular Foods (soft, moist, regularly textured foods)

Alternative Methods of Nutrition

When someone is unable to chew or swallow because of oral radiation, jaw injury, or stroke, alternative methods of nutrition may be provided to maintain proper nutritional intake. Health care professionals will work closely to ensure that these alternative methods are used correctly and safely. Whenever alternative feeding methods are used, it is important to watch closely for any signs of infection, such as pain, redness, swelling at the site of intravenous needle or feeding tube, or fever.

INTRAVENOUS FEEDING (Parenteral Nutrition):

Intravenous feeding is the process of providing nutrients directly into the blood stream. Intravenous fluid intake can be used as an eating substitute for short periods of time. It is the preferred alternative when adequate protein and calories cannot be provided by oral or other routes, or when the gastrointestinal system is not functioning. This is more commonly seen in hospital settings, and less often in nursing care or in-home settings because of increased risk of complications.

TUBE FEEDING (Enteral Nutrition):

Tube feeding is the process of inserting a flexible, narrow tube into some portion of the digestive tract and placing liquid formulas or liquefied foods into the tube to meet the person's nutritional needs. Tube feeding is used when food cannot be ingested through the mouth, but there may be a cleared passage in the esophagus and stomach, and even partial functioning of the gastrointestinal tract. Tube feeding is preferred over intravenous feeding to maintain the functioning of the intestines, provide for immunity to infection, and avoid complications related to intravenous feeding.

Resources

- Caring for the Patient with Cancer at Home: A Guide for Patients and Families from the American Cancer Society (http://www.cancer.org)

- American Medical Association Guide to Home Caregiving (http://www.ama-assn.org)

- Jackson Siegelbaum Gastroenterology Patient Information (http://www.gicare.com)

- Vanderbilt University Nutrition Clinic

- Tufts University (http://nutrition.tufts.edu/consumer/pyramid.html)

- USDA & DHHS, Dietary Guidelines for Americans, 5th ed. 2000 (http://www.usda.gov/cnpp/Pubs/DG2000)

Nutritional recipes located in "_Resources and Inventories_" Chapter.

– Respite –
Relief for the Caregiver

Caregiving is Hard; I Miss My Life

I want to help my Mom in every way that I can – it's hard to see her struggle with everyday activities. But even when I work myself to the point of exhaustion, I feel like I haven't done enough. Hiring outside help is so expensive that we can only afford eight hours of extra care per week. I need more than eight hours just to feel free -- just to be with myself and rejuvenate.

I miss the relationship I had with my Mom, when I could really be myself and she could really be herself. Now everything is so intertwined that it's hard for us to see each other clearly. I want to be friends again. I really miss that.

--- Caregiver for mother with Multiple Sclerosis

Taking care of one's self may seem almost impossible, given lack of time and/or energy. It may even feel selfish to take time for one's self. It is important to remember that we can only take as good care of others as we do of ourselves. This chapter will offer information to help you be aware of and deal with the stress and strain of caregiving.

Caregivers often feel lonely and isolated, which, in turn, can increase feelings of resentment and guilt. Common complaints include sleep disturbance, lack of appetite, upset stomach, tight chest, backaches, headaches, exhaustion, trouble concentrating, difficulty making decisions, and being argumentative, impatient, easily upset, and critical.

We have divided caregiver dynamics into three parts: feeling, dealing, and healing. Through acknowledging and understanding our own feelings, we can start dealing. With the process of dealing comes the healing.

FEELING

At any given time a caregiver may experience a wide range of emotions from anger to relief. Events and circumstances may even precipitate emotions. It is very important to acknowledge and validate your feelings, even those that seem disturbing to you. Most likely these feelings are normal.

> **IF YOUR FEELINGS EVOLVE INTO SUICIDAL OR HOMICIDAL THOUGHTS, PLEASE SPEAK TO A PROFESSIONAL OR CALL A CRISIS CENTER HOT LINE.**

The following are some emotions that you may feel:

- **ANGER:** Anger can be directed in many directions. It may be aimed toward the one you are caring for, your children, your spouse, or even towards people you don't know. It is important to deal with these feelings because anger can make the situation more stressful and can even lead to physical illnesses.

- **GRIEF:** Grief can ensue from losing your independence, the life you had (including friendships), and losing the person you knew and loved.

- **SHAME:** Shame can come from feeling like you are not doing enough or being embarrassed about the senior's behavior. You may even be ashamed of your own self-image, because you are focusing so much on the care receiver that you do not allow time to take care of yourself.

- **POWERLESSNESS:** Feeling powerless to change or control the situation.

- **SORRY FOR SELF:** It is common to feel sorry for one's self. However, try to form a more positive mindset. For example, instead of saying "Why me?", say "I am doing the best I can to care for my loved one."

- **GUILT:** Guilt can often come from feeling that you are not doing enough. Have realistic expectations and maintain balance. You can only do so much, and that is okay.

DEALING

Dealing is how you manage the stress and feelings that come with caregiving. It is acknowledging your emotional and physical state so that you can take action.

There are both positive and negative techniques in coping with a caregiving situation.

Positive methods for coping are:

- ▶ **COMMUNICATION:** Communicate your needs and wants.

- ▶ **AWARENESS:** Be aware of your emotional and physical symptoms such as moodiness, insomnia, change in weight gain/loss, illness, etc.

- ▶ **LAUGHTER:** There is scientific evidence that laughter releases stress and lowers blood pressure.

- ▶ **MEDITATION:** Meditation can help relieve stress by relaxing the body and mind and is not hard to do. The numerous benefits can help in many aspects of life.

▶ **PHYSICAL EXERCISE:** Exercise can give you more energy and help to relieve stress. Even a 15-minute walk can help.

▶ **NUTRITIOUS DIET:** Choose a variety of healthy foods. Eating regularly gives you the energy you need to maintain your health and continue in your important role as caregiver.

Negative methods for coping are:

▶ **SELF-MEDICATING:** Relying on excessive drug or alcohol intake to calm your nerves.

▶ **DENIAL AND/OR AVOIDANCE:** Instead of validating your feelings and the reality of the situation, you pretend that the feelings don't exist or that the situation is not what it is.

▶ **ADDICTIONS:** Any habit that is done in excess and for immediate gratification without consideration of consequences. Shopping, sex, and overeating are some common addictions.

HEALING

Healing is a stage of opportunity for the caregiver. The process of healing can provide the caregiver with hope and self-growth. However, the healing process is not an easy one and can be an ongoing process. Beneficial channels to start the healing process are:

▪ Clergy -- Spiritual guidance

▪ Support groups -- Sharing ideas and experiences can help you feel less isolated. These groups offer opportunities to receive help and to extend help to others.

- Learning opportunities – Attending workshops and reading literature on caregiving can promote confidence.

- Compassion – Finding outlets to help others can be very healing.

- Continue a healthy lifestyle – Include healthy eating habits, physical exercise, and meditation.

Effects of Caregiving

Adult children of aging parents may experience **role reversal**, as they've always counted on their parents to take care of themselves and also be supportive of the family unit. The entire family is affected by the caregiver's new role. For example, young children and the caregiver's spouse may feel neglected. In turn, this can cause friction and conflict for the family. The normal routine of living is interrupted on a temporary to permanent basis: The recipient of care may need to live with the caregiver, which can restrict the caregiver's social life and infringe on privacy.

There may be negative or positive feelings from both the recipient of care and the caregiver. If it was a difficult relationship before it became a caregiving situation, issues or family dynamics can often resurface. Caregivers can also experience grief related to the role reversal. It is natural for you to feel loss, because you are seeing a once-strong person, whom you have depended on, become more dependent and demanding.

Although often positive and rewarding, caregiving can take a toll on caregivers. It is important to be aware of the potentially negative health effects that can result from caregiving.

Physical Signs of Caregiver Stress:

▶ Disturbed Sleep

▶ Back, shoulder, or neck pain, muscle tension

▶ Headaches

▶ Stomach/digestive problems (upset or acid stomach, cramps, heartburn, gas, irritable bowel syndrome, constipation, diarrhea)

▶ Weight fluctuation (gain or loss)

▶ Loss of hair

▶ Fatigue

▶ High blood pressure, irregular heart beat, palpitations

▶ Chest pain

▶ Perspiration

▶ Skin disorders (hives, eczema, psoriasis, tics, itching)

▶ Periodontal disease, jaw pain

▶ Reproductive problems/infertility

▶ Weakened immune system suppression: more colds, flu, infections

▶ Sexual dysfunction/lack of libido

Emotional Signs of Caregiver Stress:

► Anxiety

► Depression

► Moodiness/mood swings

► "Butterflies"

► Irritability, frustration, road rage

► Memory problems and lack of concentration

► Feeling out of control

► Increased substance abuse

► Phobias

► Argumentativeness

► Feeling of isolation

► Job dissatisfaction

If you are experiencing some of the signs listed above, consider talking with a healthcare professional, who can help you to evaluate your situation and suggest responses. It is important that a family caregiver realize that he or she is not alone. Getting support will help reduce caregiver stress, as well as reduce the associated physical and emotional risks of ongoing stress.

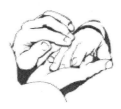

Remember, it is not selfish to focus on your own needs and desires when you are a family caregiver. In fact, it is a necessity to take initiative with your own physical and emotional care, or else it could make you less useful to the person for whom you are caring.

A SIMPLE CAREGIVER STRESS TEST

The following test will help you become aware of the emotions, pressures, and stress you currently feel. Which of the following are seldom true, sometimes true, often true, or usually true?

- I find I can't get enough sleep.

- I don't have enough time for myself.

- I don't have time to be with other family members besides the person I care for.

- I feel guilty about my situation.

- I don't get out much anymore.

- I have conflict with the person I care for.

- I have conflicts with other family members.

- I cry often.

- I worry about having enough money to make ends meet.

- I don't feel I have enough knowledge or experience to give care as well as I'd like.

- My own health is not good.

- My care receiver needs constant supervision.

- I rarely get away from my caregiving situation.

If the response to one or more of these statements is usually true or often true, it may be time to begin looking for help both in caring for the care receiver and in taking care of yourself.

TAKE CARE OF YOURSELF!

As a caregiver, it is a necessity to take care of yourself in order to take care of your loved one. Below are tips on caring for yourself:

- Incorporate activities that give you pleasure even when you don't really feel like it. Listen to music, work in the garden, engage in a hobby ... whatever you enjoy.

- Pamper yourself. Take a warm bath and light candles. Find some time for a manicure or a massage.

- Eat balanced meals to nurture your body. Find time to exercise even if it's a short walk everyday. Do the best you can to sleep at least seven hours a night.

- "Laughter is the best medicine." Buy a light-hearted book or rent a comedy video. Whenever you can, try to find some humor in everyday situations.

- Keep a journal. Write down your thoughts and feelings. This helps provide perspective on your situation and serves as a release for your emotions.

- Arrange a telephone contact with a family member, a friend, or a volunteer from a church or senior center so that someone calls each day to be sure everything is all right. This person could relieve you of responsibility by contacting other family members to let them know the status of the care receiver, or if you need anything.

■ Try to set a time for afternoons or evenings out. Seek out friends and family to help you so that you can have some time away from the home. And, if it is difficult to leave, invite friends and family over to visit with you. Share some tea or coffee. It is important that you interact with others.

■ Join a support group or seek out people who are going through the same experiences that you are living each day. If you can't leave the house, internet support groups are available.

■ Draw strength from your faith. A congregation in a church or synagogue can provide the encouragement you need to feel good about your caregiving role and may also be able to provide a break for you from time to time.

What is Respite?

Respite is a temporary break for a caregiver. It is a break from caring for someone with a disability, chronic illness, or others who need special care.

> " Respite is a needed and deserved service ... it supports family well-being "

It can be planned or emergency. A planned break can be for a few hours to go to church, to run errands, to visit with friends or other family. It can be for an evening, overnight, or a week or more for a vacation. An emergency break might be needed if you have to go to the hospital or a funeral, have a family emergency, or need to go out of town for work.

Respite can happen in your home (with you there or you could go out). It could be at someone else's home, in the community (for example the park, a movie), or at a facility (like a group home or assisted living facility). The respite provider may be someone you know, like a relative, neighbor, or friend, or you may find a provider through an agency. You and your loved one will benefit from respite.

WHO NEEDS RESPITE SERVICES?

YOU! Anyone doing caregiving needs respite services. It is necessary to have respite in order to continue doing a good job caregiving.

WHY DO PEOPLE NEED RESPITE?

Respite is meant to give relief to families from the daily, constant care of a loved one. It helps make families stronger. It is a needed and DESERVED service. Respite supports family well-being and helps prevent crisis. It provides a caregiver the opportunity to spend time with other family members or friends, to go to church, or to run errands. It can relieve and support caregivers during stressful times. It also allows the loved one to socialize outside of the family, make new friends, and enjoy new experiences.

HOW DO YOU CHOOSE A RESPITE PROVIDER?

It is important to decide what kind of respite you need. You need to decide if you want a few hours each week or one night a month. You may have to go somewhere every Saturday, or you may need an occasional weekend away. Decide if you want the respite to be provided in or out of the home. In interviewing potential respite providers, ask as many questions as you need to.

It is important that you feel comfortable with your paid respite provider.

- Tell them what activities/duties are expected.

- Discuss the days and amount of time you need, as well as the rate of pay.

- Ask about current and past employment.

- Ask for three references, including names and phone numbers.

- You may decide to do a background check. This can be done through the Tennessee State Bureau of Investigation or on the Internet.

- Ask if they have training in caring for people with the special needs of your loved one.

- Ask if they have CPR/First Aid training or certification.

- Ask if they have reliable transportation.

- If they are taking your loved one out, ask to see their driver's license.

FINANCIAL ASSISTANCE

- Alzheimer's Association

- ARC

- Family Caregiver Support Program(of the Area Agency on Aging & Disability)

- Home health, personal support and sitter services

- Relative Caregivers Programs

- FiftyForward Respite Caregivers/Senior Companions

VOLUNTEER PROGRAMS

- Respite Caregivers

- Some congregations informally

- Some neighborhoods informally

ADULT DAY CARE -- TRADITIONAL

- Knowles Home Adult Day Services

- Catholic Charities Adult Day Program

- Centennial Adultcare Center

- FiftyForward Adult Day Services

- Some assisted living facilities offer day services as well

OVERNIGHT (Typically there is a minimum stay)

- Many assisted living and nursing facilities offer overnight stays.
  Sometimes they will offer it at no charge as an orientation.

- Veterans Administration

OTHER ASSISTANCE

- Local senior centers

- Mental Health Association

- County Social Services Departments

- Volunteer programs through churches, senior agencies, universities.

To talk with someone about your specific needs and to find what community service is right for you, call your local ADRC (Aging and Disability Resource Connection) or Area Agency on Aging and Disability (AAAD).

Caregiver's Bill of Rights

AS A CAREGIVER, I HAVE THE RIGHT ...

- To take care of myself—to rest when I'm tired, to eat well, and to take breaks from caregiving when I need them.

- To recognize the limits of my own endurance and strength.

- To seek help from family, involved parties, and the community at large.

- To socialize, maintain my interests, and to do the things I enjoy.

- To acknowledge my feelings, whether positive or negative, including frustration, anger, and depression; and to express them constructively.

- To take pride in the valuable work I do, and to applaud the courage and inventiveness it takes to meet the needs of my care recipient.

-- Author Unknown

Working with Employers

> *There are only four kinds of people in this world ...*
>
> *Those who have been caregivers*
>
> *Those who currently are caregivers*
>
> *Those who will be caregivers*
>
> *Those who will need caregivers.*
>
> ~ Rosalynn Carter, 1997

Caregivers come in many forms and have many different circumstances. Those caregivers who also have an outside job will often find themselves torn between their work responsibilities and those of caring for their older adult. This is true whether the caregiving is in the senior's home, in the caregiver's home, in a facility, or long-distance. In the 1980s American businesses adapted their human resource policies to accommodate the needs of workers with young children. Now many of those same workers face a new responsibility: providing care for an older parent, relative, or friend.

For a variety of reasons it is important that you let the human resource department at your place of employment know of your situation. If your performance is not up to previous levels because of time spent with caregiving, it is better for your employer to know this than to assume that you just don't care about your job. The HR professional may know of help that the employer can provide or may have a list of resources.

Begin by being honest—you want to be a good employee and a good caregiver. Ask if your employer has any eldercare programs. If not, help the manager understand what is required of you as a caregiver and be prepared to MAKE A CREATIVE PROPOSAL ON HOW YOU CAN FULFILL YOUR ROLES AS CAREGIVER AND AS GOOD EMPLOYEE.

Some solutions are:

- Flexible hours

- Working from home

- Cafeteria-style benefits that allow you to choose adult day care, etc. instead of some other benefits (such as child care) that you do not need

- Talking to others at the job site with similar caregiver issues

- Learning about resources that can help balance job and caregiving

Some employers may not have faced this issue with an employee before, and they will need to be educated about the effects of caregiving on employees. This is particularly true of younger managers who have not yet faced the issue in their own families. Some employers assume that Medicare pays for every senior service and do not understand the work interruptions or absenteeism for doctors' visits or other crises.

Your caregiving role may mean that you make difficult decisions regarding advancement, travel, hours, etc. The key is to balance your personal needs, your family's needs, your senior's needs, and your employment responsibilities.

COUNCIL ON
AGING

Leaving Home

When the family home seems too big, too hard to manage, with too many steps or too much yard, the question becomes where to go next. It is advisable to do some preliminary work by asking friends for recommendations before a crisis arises. Many families must make these decisions within a few days of an unexpected hospital stay.

When the worsening condition of a senior who chose to remain at home with or without additional help, requires a move to an assisted living facility or nursing home, a physician and/or a family caregiver may be the one to initiate this decision. This can be a very traumatic occasion for the senior, but the facility's staff can be helpful.

Cultural and Ethnic Diversity in Long-Term Care

America is more diverse now than ever before, including both the people needing long-term care and the people providing that care. Whether services are provided in a home or in a facility, your loved one will be interacting with people of different lifestyles, races, cultures, economic backgrounds, and religions.

Facility care will probably be provided by people from a variety of cultures. Also, the other people receiving care in these settings are more diverse than in the past. It is important to ask about religious practices and tolerance, food, activities, language and even the music played, to find out whether your loved one will be comfortable in the facility. The level of formality at a facility can also affect how satisfied he/she will be. If your loved one is physically frail but mentally alert, you'll need to ask about the functioning levels of other residents and how they interact with each other.

Senior Housing Definitions

■ **Independent Living:** A residential setting for senior adults that may or may not provide supportive services. Under this living arrangement, the senior adult leads an independent lifestyle that requires minimal or no extra assistance. In some settings units are owned; in others, they are rented. Generally referred to as elderly housing in the government-subsidized environment, independent living may also include rental-assisted or market rate apartments or cottages, where residents usually have complete choice in whether to participate in a facility's services or programs.

■ **Continuing Care Retirement Community:** A continuing care retirement community (CCRC) offers several levels of housing and services that may include independent living, assisted living, and/or nursing home care. A CCRC offers independent living in an apartment or duplex with an array of supportive services such as transportation, meals, housekeeping services, and exercise classes, as well as access to health care in adjoining assisted living and nursing home facilities. A CCRC is different from other housing and care facilities for seniors because it usually entails a written agreement or contract between the resident (frequently lasting the term of the resident's lifetime) and the community, which provides the continuum of housing, services, and a health care system, commonly all on one campus or site. Depending on the level of assistance needed, an individual may move throughout the community. It is best to make the decision to enter a CCRC while one is still healthy and active. Waiting for an "event" to happen may make it difficult for a new resident to adjust and/or feel happy in the new surroundings.

Most important, a CCRC offers companionship and the social support of a variety of people. When and if the time comes for more care, the senior is still part of the same community.

■ **Assisted Care Living Facilities:** A licensed residential setting that offers a variety of support services such as meals, housekeeping, activities, transportation, and assistance with bathing, dressing, and medication. Be sure the services provided meet the specific needs of the resident. This is a broad category of housing, and not every assisted living facility provides all of the services. In Tennessee there is another category of licensed housing called Homes for the Aged that, unlike ACLFs, are not required to offer licensed medical care.

■ **Nursing Home (sometimes called Healthcare Centers):** Patients generally rely on assistance for most or all daily living activities (such as bathing, dressing, and toileting). Provides 24-hour licensed skilled nursing care (Level II) for the more acute patients. Intermediate care (Level I) is a less intensive level of care than skilled nursing care and may also be offered. Nursing homes may provide care by nurses, physical therapists, speech therapists, or occupational therapists. Some facilities have secure units and special care for individuals who are memory-impaired.

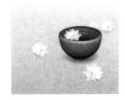

Senior Housing Shopping Guidelines

If you are seeking a residence for someone who cannot visit the residence personally, it is important to respect his/her needs and wishes by including the senior in the process as much as possible. The result will be greater satisfaction.

The following are shopping guidelines for reviewing important services in assisted living communities. Many apply to nursing homes and continuing care retirement communities also. Make several visits at various times of day to each residence you are considering.

Atmosphere

- As you tour the residence, is the décor attractive and homelike?

- Did you receive a warm greeting from staff welcoming you to the residence?

- Does the administrator/staff call residents by name and interact warmly with them as you tour the residence?

- Do residents socialize with each other and appear happy and comfortable?

- Are you able to talk with residents about how they like the residence and staff?

- Would the residents seem to be appropriate housemates for your loved one?

- Are staff members appropriately dressed, personable, and outgoing?

- Do the staff members treat each other in a professional manner?

- Are visits with the resident welcomed at any time?

Physical Features

- Is the community well designed for residents' needs?

- Are doorways, hallways, and rooms accommodating to wheelchairs and walkers?

- Are handrails available to aid in walking?

- Are cupboards and shelves easy to reach?

- Are floors of a non-skid material and carpets firm for safe walking?

- Does the residence have good natural and artificial lighting?

- Is the residence clean, free of odors and appropriately heated/cooled?

- Does the residence meet local and/or state licensing requirements?

- Does the residence have sprinklers and clearly marked exits?

- Does the residence have a means of security if a resident wanders?

Needs Assessments, Contracts, Costs, and Finances

- Is a contractual agreement available that discloses healthcare and supportive services, all fees, as well as admission and discharge provisions?

- Is there a written plan for the care of each resident?

- Does the residence have a process for assessing a potential resident's need for services, and are those needs addressed periodically?

- Does this process include the resident, the family, and facility staff along with the potential resident's physician?

- When may a contract be terminated, and what are refund policies?

■ Are additional services available if the resident's needs change?

■ Is there a procedure to pay for additional services, like nursing care, when the services are needed on a temporary basis?

■ Are there different costs for various levels or categories of services?

■ Are residents required to purchase renters' insurance for their personal property?

■ Is staff available to meet scheduled and unscheduled needs?

■ Is there an appeals process for dissatisfied residents?

Medication and Health Care

■ Does the residence have specific policies regarding storage of medication, assistance with medications, training and supervision of staff, and record keeping?

■ Is self-administration of medication allowed?

■ Is there a staff person to coordinate visits from a nurse, physical therapist, occupational therapist, etc. if needed?

■ Are staff members available to assist residents who experience memory, orientation, or judgment losses?

■ Does a physician, nurse practitioner, or nurse visit regularly for medical checkups?

■ Does the residence have a clearly-stated procedure for responding to a resident's medical emergency?

■ To what extent are medical services available and how are they provided?

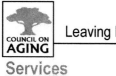
Services

- Is staff available to provide 24-hour assistance with activities of daily living (ADLs) if needed? ADLs include: dressing, eating, mobility, hygiene, grooming, bathing, toileting, incontinence care, using the telephone, shopping, and laundry.

- Does the residence provide housekeeping services in residents' units?

- Does the residence provide transportation to doctors' offices, the hairdresser, shopping, and other activities desired by residents?

- Can residents arrange for transportation on fairly short notice?

- Are pharmacy, barber/beautician and/or therapy services offered on-site?

Individual Unit Features

- Are units for single and double occupancy available?

- Do residents have their own lockable doors?

- Is a 24-hour emergency response system accessible from the unit?

- Are bathrooms private, and are they accessible for wheelchairs and walkers?

- Are residents able to bring their own furnishings for their unit, and what may they bring? What is provided?

- Do all units have a telephone and cable TV, and how is billing handled?

- Is a kitchen area/unit provided with a refrigerator, sink, and cooking element?

- May residents keep food in their units?

- May residents smoke in their units? In public areas?

- May residents decorate their own units?

Social & Recreational Activities

- Is there evidence of an organized activities program, such as a posted daily schedule, events in progress, reading materials, visitors, etc.?

- Do residents participate in activities outside of the residence in the neighboring community?

- Do volunteers come into the residence to help with or conduct programs?

- Does the residence create a sense of community by requiring residents to participate in certain activities or to perform simple chores for the group as a whole?

- Are residents' pets allowed in the residence? Who is responsible for their care?

- Are any religious services available at the residence?

Food Service

- Does the residence provide three nutritionally balanced meals a day, seven days a week?

- Are snacks available? Is water or juice offered several times in between meals?

- May residents request special foods?

- Are common dining areas available?

- May residents eat meals in their units?

- May meals be provided at a time a resident likes, or are there set times for meals?

- Ask about having a meal at the residence. Is the food tasty? Do the residents seem to enjoy mealtime? Are there a variety of choices?

-- Source: AFLA Web Site 2002

Questions to Ask an Administrator or Social Worker

When you visit a facility, ask to see the state survey results. This inspection report must be made available to those who ask. Other tips:

- Ask about the staffing ratio.

- Ask if the administrator is licensed as well as the facility.

- Ask about smoke detectors, sprinklers, and fire and other emergency drills.

- Ask about the residents council, how often it meets and what it does.

- Ask if the nursing home is Medicare-certified and Medicaid-certified.

- Ask how many residents each CNA (certified nursing assistant) works with.

- Ask if the facility has corrected all deficiencies from its last inspection report.

- Ask how many staff members are on duty for each shift.

- Ask to see the facility's Resident Bill of Rights.

Downsizing and Moving

It is always difficult to leave a long-loved home, but doing so in good health and with the aid of children, relatives, and other services can make moving much less stressful.

> **It is important that the senior be a part of the process as much as he or she desires and as health allows.**

Before the need arises, loved ones should explore each other's expectations about downsizing. They need to be realistic about how much to move into smaller spaces, and should express their wishes regarding family heirlooms. Some families have such talks, but seldom explore the overwhelming task of emptying the house!

Many of us will be called upon to downsize and liquidate our parents' things. Making a decision about what's to be done with the personal property of someone you love is a complicated and emotional task. The need to downsize or liquidate often means vacating "a home place"-- the place where children grew up.

The thought of clearing away clothing, personal papers, photos, furniture, hand-made holiday decorations, personal items, tools, linens, your own baby clothes and collections is reason enough to ignore the chore. And many people react by doing nothing. Some attack the chore and make decisions far too quickly to suit everyone involved. The options for completing the task include: **distribute, donate, discard,** or **sell.**

Expect to be overwhelmed by the memories evoked as you uncover photos, toys, and mementoes. Accept the help of friends and family.

Don't try to do the whole house at once. Set a smaller goal like a room, a cupboard, or a closet. If you find a box or area of small items that you want to take time to examine, box it and do it later. Remove the things that will go with their owner or to family and friends.

Start at the back corner of the room by removing the fluff (the broken or useless items) and arranging the items to be examined and appraised. Focus on one area at a time; just do it in small portions at a time. With every visit to the house -- even to set the thermostat or look for some papers, try to clear away some trash. Junk mail and medical paperwork can pile up quickly. Clutter can smother your mission. Simply clearing a table top can improve your attitude the next time you walk into the house.

After you have determined which items will be distributed, donated, discarded, and sold, act on the decisions. Gather family, selected friends, and heirs for the purpose of division and distribution. Have things picked up by non-profit agencies or discarded properly. Soon, the end of the job will seem attainable.

You may choose to hire an expert for sorting, pricing, selling, moving, and staging. Professionals like realtors, senior move managers, family advisors, and geriatric care managers can help find a service. Examine your abilities and discuss your requirements with friends who have had similar experiences. Having a downsizing and/or liquidation sale from the site allows you the option *not to sell* as the day progresses. But there may be items left after the sale is through. An auction sale moves more quickly with little room for indecision. But an auction will *clear the space* in a day.

Seniors may be more agreeable to giving up some items (silver, furniture, heirlooms) if they are being given to grandchildren or special friends or neighbors. For keepsakes, including pictures, ask for the senior's input in labeling for future generations.

Senior Move Managers

For people contemplating or facing the daunting task of transition and downsizing from a long-held single-family home, there are support agencies available today. This new industry group, known as "Senior Mover Managers," has gained footing in the last ten years. Typical services may include:

Guidance on area communities, realtor referral, customized floor plans

Preparation for selling the current house, organizing, de-cluttering, sorting, clearing, packing up, storing household goods, cleaning up

Coordinating the move, arranging/supervising movers and the moving process

Turn-key set up of the new residence, interfacing with family and other professionals

Arranging for the profitable disposal of unwanted items through estate sales, donation, or consignment.

Contact the National Association of Senior Move Managers (online at http://www.nasmm.com) for a list of local companies. Senior information and referral centers can also link you to local resources.

End-of-Life Issues

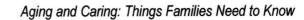

Palliative Care

Palliative care is a concept, and it is a service. Palliative care aims to relieve suffering and to improve quality of life for patients with advanced or terminal illness. It also addresses the needs of families of these patients. Palliative care is provided by an interdisciplinary team and is offered in conjunction with other forms of medical treatment.

Palliative care programs include a variety of resources—medical and nursing specialists, social workers, and clergy—to deliver the highest quality of care to patients with advanced illness. Vigorous pain and symptom control is a part of all stages of treatment.

The palliative care approach decreases the length of hospital and ICU stays and eases patient transitions between care settings, resulting in increased patient and family satisfaction. Successful palliative care programs use an array of delivery systems, from consultative services to inpatient units.

Hospice

Do not quit reading this section because of the word "Hospice." If there is one statement that has been said many times over, it is this: "I wish I had called earlier."

WHAT IS HOSPICE CARE?

Hospice is special end-of-life care for people with life-limiting illnesses, as well as a way to support their loved ones. A type of care, rather than a specific place of care, it focuses on comfort rather than cure. It neither

> " *Hospice care is a type of care ... that focuses on comfort rather than cure.* "

accelerates nor postpones a person's death. Additional services include partnership with health care professionals and educational initiatives. The mission is to provide care, so that each person can live each day as fully as possible with dignity, comfort, and peace.

WHO IS HOSPICE CARE FOR?

Hospice serves those who have illnesses that can no longer be cured. Care is provided for patients with a variety of illnesses, including but not limited to: end-stage dementia, congestive heart failure, end-stage Parkinson's disease, chronic obstructive pulmonary disease, ALS (Lou Gehrig's Disease), cancer, AIDS, and other end-stage chronic diseases. A person is eligible for hospice care when life expectancy is 12 months or less.

WHAT DOES HOSPICE DO TO HELP PATIENTS WITH LIFE-LIMITING ILLNESSES?

Hospice, together with a patient's physician, helps manage a patient's physical symptoms and pain, allowing him or her to live more fully and with dignity. Hospice also helps ease the emotional burden that patients and their loved ones may have, thereby increasing the quality of the time they have together.

WHAT DOES HOSPICE DO TO HELP CAREGIVERS AND OTHER FAMILY MEMBERS?

Hospice social service specialists offer emotional support and resources to cope during this difficult process. Hospice delivers medications and equipment, assists with personal care needs such as baths, and helps with practical matters such as running errands or relieving the caregiver for needed time away. Often, what is needed most is simply a kind ear and experienced guidance on what to expect. Hospice also offers bereavement counseling, so that family and friends can prepare for the loss and manage their grief.

WHO IS A PART OF THE HOSPICE CARE TEAM?

The patient and his or her loved ones are at the center of the hospice team. Patients and caregivers are supported by a team that works with each patient to help manage the pain and control the symptoms associated with illness and to provide personal, respectful care. Hospice team members include:

▶ **Medical Director:** The Director oversees the care plan and consults regularly with other team members. The Medical Director also works with the patient's primary physician.

▶ **Nurses:** Hospice nurses provide compassionate and skilled nursing care. They work closely with the physician to manage pain and symptoms, individualize patient care, and inform and support the patient's loved ones.

▶ **Social Service Professionals:** Experienced social service professionals nurture and care for the patients' and families' emotional needs through all stages of the illness. They provide counseling and assistance with a variety of areas including, but not limited to, social and economic needs, advance directives (such as living wills), Medicare/Medicaid and Supplemental Security Income information, and funeral arrangements.

▶ **Home Health Aides:** Home health aides provide personal care and comfort for patients by assisting with cleanliness and the safety and emotional support of the patient.

▶ **Spiritual Counselor:** Clergy members offer spiritual guidance and support. They assist the patient's minister, rabbi, or other spiritual representative in whatever capacity chosen. They also can conduct funeral services, if requested.

▶ **Volunteers:** Volunteers are specially screened and trained to provide companionship and assistance to patients during the last stages of their illnesses.

▶ **Bereavement Experts:** Hospice may have licensed mental health professionals offering bereavement assistance to survivors following the death of their loved one. Individual and family counseling and support groups are available as well. Support is extended to family members for as long as 13 months after a loss.

AT WHAT POINT SHOULD WE INVOLVE HOSPICE?

A person can enter a hospice program of care when a physician believes life expectancy is 12 months or less. While many people believe that hospice care is unavailable or inappropriate until a patient reaches the last days of his life, there is actually much that can be done many months earlier to enhance one's quality of life. Pain and symptom management, emotional support and guidance, assistance in organizing a patient's affairs, and support for caregivers and loved ones are just a few of the many benefits available well before the end of life. Entering a program of hospice care earlier also allows more time for a person to consider his choices and to make his wishes known to loved ones. Such forethought relieves the caregivers of making difficult decisions on their own.

HOW DO I BECOME ENROLLED IN A PROGRAM OF HOSPICE CARE?

Patients need a referral from a physician consenting to work with the hospice team. Anyone can make the initial referral to the program, including the patient, family members, clergy, a hospital discharge planner, or the interdisciplinary team of a long-term care or assisted living facility.

HOW IS HOSPICE CARE PAID FOR?

Most people have Medicare, Medicaid, or private insurance that covers the cost of hospice services.

WHAT IF MY LOVED ONE IS NOT QUITE READY TO ENTER A PROGRAM OF HOSPICE CARE?

Hospice is happy to provide information about all of the services available. The staff will be happy to help you learn more about how hospice can work to meet your specific needs at any point in the course of care. Hospice care acknowledges that patients and their families are always in complete control of their own choices and decisions.

WHAT HOSPICES ARE AVAILABLE?

Ask your doctor, your hospital social worker or case manager, your friends, or look in the phone book or the Council on Aging's *Directory of Services for Seniors.*

Funeral Planning

Thinking ahead can help you make informed and thoughtful decisions about funeral arrangements. It allows you to choose the specific items wanted and compare the prices offered by several funeral providers. It also spares caregivers the stress of making these decisions under the pressure of time and emotions. Arrangements can be made directly with a funeral establishment or through a funeral planning or memorial society.

An important consideration is where the remains will be buried, entombed, or scattered. This too should be discussed and planned well in advance. It is a good idea to review your decision every few years.

Many people prearrange their funerals and prepay some or all of the expenses involved. This may take the form of an insurance policy specifically to pay costs connected to the funeral and burial. State law on this subject varies from state to state, as does consumer protection.

Some points to consider are:

- What are you paying for—merchandise like a casket and vault or funeral services as well?

- What happens to the money you've prepaid? What happens to the interest income on money that is prepaid and put into a trust account?

- Are you protected if the firm you dealt with goes out of business?

- Can you cancel the contract and get a refund?

- What happens if you move to a different area of the country?

- Make plans in advance to choose a burial plot, columbarium, or mausoleum.

- *Funeral homes must disclose the cost of all goods and services and, upon request, provide a written price list for your review.*

- Organ and body donations <u>must</u> also be preplanned during the person's lifetime.

- Plans should be placed in writing and kept where they can be easily found by family members. It is important that family members be told that such plans exist.

- The Social Security Administration, the Veterans Administration, and life and casualty insurance companies pay death benefits. Call these agencies to determine coverage and benefits.

- The Veterans Administration offers many benefits for honorably discharged veterans. Veterans and their spouses and children may be buried in veterans' cemeteries. Arrangements should be made through a local funeral director. Veterans may receive money for a private burial and a headstone at no charge. Information on other veterans' programs can be obtained by calling 1-800-827-1000 or write Department of Veterans Affairs, 810 Vermont Avenue NW, Washington, D.C. 20420 for the booklet, "Free Benefits for Veterans and Dependents." To access benefits, you may need a copy of the honorable discharge. This can be obtained from the National Personnel Record Center, 9700 Page Avenue, St. Louis, Missouri 63132 or online at http://www.va.gov.

End of Life Signs and Symptoms

ONE TO THREE MONTHS

- Withdrawal from the world and people

- Decreased food intake

- Increase in sleep

- Going inside of self

- Less communication

ONE TO TWO WEEKS

- Agitation

- Talking with the unseen

- Confusion

- Picking at clothes

- Decreased blood pressure

- Pulse increase or decrease

- Color changes -- pale, bluish

- Increased perspiration

- Respiration irregularities

- Congestion

- Complaints of body being tired and heavy

- Not eating, taking few fluids

- Body temperature, hot/cold

DAYS OR HOURS

- Intensification of One to Two Week signs (see previous page)

- Surge of energy

- Decrease in blood pressure

- Eyes glassy, tearing, half open

- Irregular breathing, stop/start

- Restlessness or no activity

- Purplish or blotchy knees, feet, hands

- Pulse weak and hard to find

- Decreased urine output

- Incontinence, may wet or stool the bed

MINUTES

- "Fish out of water" breathing

- Cannot be awakened

At the Time of Death

- If a death occurs at home, call the Emergency Medical Service for your area or the Police Department. If under hospice care, you may call your hospice nurse. If you are certain the person is dead, call the Police Department. These professionals will tell you what to do next.

- Contact your minister/ rabbi and your funeral director and immediate family members. Your religious advisor will provide not only comfort but also planning for a service or memorial.

- Some funeral directors will help with the obituary and provide the death certificate. Additional certified copies of the death certificate will be needed as you settle the estate.

- Have a friend watch your home during the visitation and funeral service. Thieves have been known to read the obituaries to learn when homes may be empty.

- Have a pad and pen readily available to note those friends who call or bring food or flowers to your home. This will help in remembering these kindnesses and thanking the giver.

Next Steps

1. Do not make snap decisions or feel pressured to make any decisions. You can always say, "I want my advisor to review that."

2. If the deceased was employed or was retired with a company's life or health insurance, call to determine benefits.

3. If a credit card was solely in the name of the deceased, notify the company and cancel the card.

4. Contact the Social Security Administration at 1-800-772-1213, and notify them of the death. You will need the Social Security number of the deceased. Some funeral homes will contact the Social Security Administration for you. In turn, SSA will notify the Centers for Medicare and Medicaid Services. If the deceased was receiving Social Security benefits at the time of death, do not cash any checks received after the death.

5. Find a copy of any insurance policies and notify the company of the death. Ask what paperwork you will need to complete. The sooner you apply for benefits, the sooner you will receive them.

6. Cancel medical, disability, and long-term care insurance that was solely for the deceased.

7. You will need several documents as you progress in settling the estate. If you do not know where all of these documents are kept, some typical places to look are: "special box" or hiding place, desk, safe deposit box, and automobile glove compartment. Some papers that may help you identify assets and liabilities are bank statements (checking and savings), tax returns, brokerage statements, and correspondence with prior employers.

8. Survivor benefits may be available from the Social Security Administration, the Veterans Administration at 1-800-827-1000, and from job pensions. You will need to apply formally.

9. Generally, federal and/or state estate/inheritance tax returns must be filed and taxes paid within nine months of a death.

10. Write down what needs to be done, who and when you contacted people, and keep all of the papers and information together in a folder or a binder. <u>Make copies of important papers and any original documents before giving them to an advisor.</u>

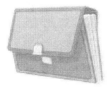

Grief

Grief is a normal and necessary process. It is how we learn to live around the hole in our heart after the loss of someone we love. Grief is work. It requires that we labor through the emotional storm of realizing loss, of saying goodbye, of being angry and alone, and of finally moving forward and rebuilding our relationship with life.

In the face of loss, you may experience:

▶ Shock/confusion

▶ Panic/crying spells

▶ Anger/guilt/relief

▶ Appetite or sleep disturbances

▶ Aimlessness

Though each of us experiences loss in our own unique way, there are similarities in this complex experience, and there are supports to help us as we journey through the wilderness. Healing begins when you:

▶ Are patient with yourself

▶ Share your feelings

▶ Pay attention to your physical needs

▶ Learn more about grief and its effects

▶ Ask for help when needed

Grief Support Groups

Grief counselors and support groups offer the opportunity to share our feelings and stories with others, to learn that there is light on the other side of grief, and to know that we are not alone. Grief counselors and support groups can be found through:

- Hospice

- Some funeral homes

- Your Church/Congregation

- Gilda's Club

- Alzheimer's Association

Manifestations of Normal Grief

Normal grief is not just sadness or depression. It reaches into every part of your life and touches your work, your relationships with others, and your image of yourself. You can expect grief to affect your feelings and your ability to think clearly. Grief may even produce unusual physical sensations and behaviors.

FEELINGS

- Sadness -- often through crying

- Anger -- sense of frustration at not being able to prevent death

- Guilt and self-reproach

- Anxiety -- from insecurity to panic attack

- Loneliness

- Fatigue -- apathy or listlessness

- Helplessness -- akin to anxiety

- Shock -- immediately after death, especially sudden death

- Yearning/pining

- Emancipation -- common after death of ambivalent relationship

- Relief -- death after a lingering illness (often accompanied by guilt)

- Numbness -- nature's way of anesthetizing survivors immediately after death

PHYSICAL SENSATIONS

- Hollowness in the stomach

- Over-sensitivity to noise

- Breathlessness, feeling short of breath

- Lack of energy

- Tightness in chest or throat

- Sense of depersonalization

- Weakness in the muscles

- Dry mouth

THOUGHT PATTERNS

■ Disbelief -- "It didn't happen"or "I'll wake up and find it was a dream."

■ Confusion -- difficulty remembering or concentrating

■ Preoccupation -- intrusive thoughts of images of the dead person

■ Sense of presence -- deceased is somehow in your current time and space

■ Hallucinations -- both visual and auditory

BEHAVIORS

■ Sleep disturbances -- difficulty going to sleep or early morning awakening

■ Appetite disturbances -- more frequently under-eating, but also overeating

■ Absent-mindedness -- doing atypical or potentially harmful things

■ Social withdrawal --loss of interest in outside world

■ Dreams of the deceased -- usually reassuring

■ Avoiding reminders of the deceased -- avoidance of grief triggers

■ Searching and calling out – may or may not be verbalized

■ Sighing -- similar to breathlessness

■ Restless overactivity -- avoiding thoughts and situations

■ Crying -- liquid emotion

■ Carrying reminders of the deceased -- pictures or items for security

■ Treasuring objects of the deceased -- wearing clothes or carrying amulets

It is normal to feel emotional pain or grief after the death of a loved one. Healing begins when you express your feelings, are patient with yourself, stay alert to your physical needs, learn more about grief and its effects, and ask for help when needed.

There are several agencies that a grieving loved one can access which provide counseling and assist in the grief process. This assistance is accomplished in individual and group settings with adults, children, preteens, teens, families, friends, and co-workers. Some grief counseling agencies are free, and others have a fee. Your congregation may also have experience in helping with grief.

Resources

Many hospices offer grief support services to individuals in Davidson and surrounding counties. They have professional grief counselors and trained volunteers to help guide you through the process of mourning.

- Alive Hospice offers free individual counseling to client families and to others on a sliding scale fee. All group sessions are free-of-charge. Call Grief Line (615) 963-4732.

- Gilda's Club provides support groups, workshops, and social events for people who suffer loss through cancer. Call (615) 329-1124. Website: http://www.gildasclub.org or in Nashville, http://www.gildasclubnashville.org

- The Center to Advance Palliative Care
  – http://www.capc.org

- National Hospice and Palliative Care Organization
  - http://www.nhpco.org

- U.S. Department of Veterans Affairs   1-800-827-1000

- Davidson County Medical Examiner   (615) 743-1800

ORGAN DONATION

- Tennessee Donor Services (information)   1-888-234-4399

BODY DONATION

- Vanderbilt Medical School   (615) 322-7948
- Meharry Medical School   1-800-386-3239

COUNSELING/SUPPORT GROUPS

Check with your congregation, and ask if a Parish Nurse, Stephen's Minister, or support group is available.

Counseling may be available at funeral homes and hospices.

Pastoral Counseling Centers of Tennessee, Inc.

Brentwood	(615) 370-9545
Clarksville	(931) 648-9009
Franklin	(615) 790-1539
Hendersonville	(615) 338-4171
Murfreesboro	(615) 904-8623
Nashville	(615) 383-0792

Subsidized Services

Subsidized Services

Some services are beyond the financial reach of many older adults. Families may be limited by how much financial support they can provide while also caring for their immediate families. In addition, parents may not feel comfortable accepting financial assistance from their family.

There are services that are provided on a sliding scale or at no charge to seniors; however, some local, state and federal programs may have long waiting lists.

Congregations can often provide help with services such as transportation, visitation, and meals by using volunteers. Congregations with a Parish Nursing and Health Ministries or Stephen Ministers program may provide some additional health services.

> **All of the services mentioned below are included in the Council on Aging's *Directory of Services for Seniors*. This information is also available online at http://www.councilonaging-midtn.org and from the Aging & Disability Resource Center's information and referral line at (615) 255-1010 or 1-877-973-6467. For services in other parts of the country, call the Eldercare Locator at 1-800-677-1116.**

ADULT DAY CARE

Private businesses, senior centers, non-profit agencies, congregations, and local governmental agencies offer adult day care. Several offer fees on a sliding scale; others accept clients receiving support through the *Veterans Administration* or the *Family Caregiver Support Program* of the *Area Agency on Aging & Disability*.

ASSESSMENT OF NEEDS

Determining precisely what services are needed is often the first step to obtaining those services. The *Area Agency on Aging & Disability* through the *Options for Community Living*, the *Medicaid/ Tenncare Waiver Program*, and the *Family Caregiver Program* all offer service coordination and some services. Agencies providing assistance with assessment, case management, and counseling include *Jewish Family Services*, the *Shepherd's Center of Madison*, *St. Luke's Family Resource Center* and the *Living at Home Coalition* operating at Catholic Charities, and the *Knowles Center*, the *Martin Center*, and the *Madison Station Senior Center of Fifty Forward*.

FINANCIAL HELP WITH FOOD, CLOTHING, UTILITIES, RENT, AND PRESCRIPTIONS

Many agencies offer financial help with the costs of everyday living; unfortunately, the help is very limited and is not offered on a continuing basis. Some agencies serve particular areas or zip codes.

FOOD SERVICES

The federal *Older Americans Act* authorizes two types of programs: home delivered meals (*Meals on Wheels*) and nutrition sites. Most delivered meals are offered at lunch five days per week. The on-site meals are also offered weekdays at lunch. In some cases participants can be picked up and brought to the site. The on-site meals also provide an opportunity for socialization with other seniors. In Middle Tennessee both of these programs are coordinated by *Mid-Cumberland Human Resource Agency* (850-3910) and Metro Social Services (880-2292). In addition some congregations organize meal delivery to seniors. Some programs may charge a small fee or ask for a donation. Check with your county health department to learn if seniors are eligible for the Commodity Supplemental Food Program. In addition, diabetic supplements and nutritional supplements (such as Ensure) may be available for no charge to low-income persons.

HEALTH SERVICES

The Legal and Financial Chapter of this book discusses programs that can help seniors pay for deductibles and co-payment connected with Medicare. Seniors should remember to take advantage of the fact that Medicare will pay for flu shots each year. County Health Departments vary in what services they provide—some provide blood pressure checks, physical exams, and dental services at little or no charge. Non-profit clinics often serve low-income persons. Hospice care is reimbursed by Medicare and many private insurance plans.

Assistance with prescription costs is now part of Medicare Part D. The State Health Insurance Assistance Program in each state (SHIP) can help families decide on an appropriate plan. In Tennessee the number is 1-877-801-0044. In addition some pharmaceutical companies provide free or reduced price medicines. Ask the physician's office for information. Veterans are eligible for special help and should contact the Veterans Administration.

HOME CARE SERVICES

There are many businesses that provide services such as sitters, homemakers, help with cooking, bathing, etc. These can be expensive. However, if there is long-term care insurance, the policy may pay for these services. The Area Agency on Aging and Disabilities coordinates several governmental programs providing some of these services. Call the Aging & Disability Resource Center (615) 255-1010 to learn the details.

Parachutes, Inc. is a local nonprofit organization that helps identify potential hazards and implement safety measures for the physically and financially challenged. Services may include deadbolt locks, smoke detectors, and furnace inspection. Call (615) 650-9877.

HOUSING

Sometimes seniors are able to remain relatively independent if they are part of a senior housing complex. Socialization with other seniors and perhaps some transportation can provide a bridge between living alone in their own home and institutionalization. The Department of Housing and Urban Development offers Section 8 housing at some residences exclusively for seniors. This means the resident pays 30 percent of his/ her income as rent, which usually includes utilities. These high-rise apartments are operated by the local housing authority or by non-profit groups such as religious denominations.

Help with the weatherization of existing homes is available through the Metropolitan Development & Housing Agency at (615) 252-8500 and the Mid-Cumberland Community Action Agencies in counties outside of Davidson. This help can take the form of grants or loans to cover home repair, including broken glass and weatherization through insulation, caulking, and weather stripping as well as wrapping water heaters and pipes and installing smoke alarms and window screens.

Assisted living can be costly. In Nashville, the Joseph B. Knowles Home (operated by the Metro Hospital Authority) and Mary, Queen of Angels both provide some sliding scale assisted living.

Nursing homes can accept private pay, Medicare, and Medicaid, but they are not required to accept all. There are many variables in terms of what particular circumstances each program covers. The Legal Aid Society (615) 244-6610 has excellent information on this subject.

LEGAL ASSISTANCE

Both the Murfreesboro Bar Association and the Nashville Bar Association offer assistance over the phone for simple legal problems. These contacts can be a way to learn if your problem requires professional legal advice. The Free Legal Clinic in Murfreesboro is on Thursday nights, and the Dial-a-Lawyer

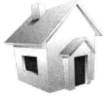

Program in Nashville is on the first Tuesday evening of each month. The Legal Aid Society also has materials, phone advice, and assistance available free of charge. They are very knowledgeable on Medicare, Social Security, and Social Security Disability.

One question a family member may have is whether to become a conservator for a relative. This means being appointed by the court to legally make decisions concerning the care of an incapacitated adult. There are several agencies which will act as a conservator for seniors; some do this on a sliding scale.

UTILITY COMPANY ASSISTANCE

Different utility companies provide varying assistance: financial assistance, resolving problems resulting from the due date of the utility bill versus the receipt of one's Social Security check, budget billing to provide equal billing throughout the year, third-party notification (where a designated relative can receive notice prior to cutoff for non-payment), and payment of the bill through bank draft.

SENIOR AND COMMUNITY CENTERS

These centers offer many activities, and most are free or have a very small charge. Meals, health screenings, care management services, wellness programs, entertainment, phone reassurance programs, and transportation are typical services.

TRANSPORTATION (See Transportation Chapter)

Senior centers sometimes offer transportation to medical appointments and shopping. Transit systems offer seniors with disabilities special transportation for a small fee.

Congregations are often a good resource for transportation when seniors need someone to help them in and out of their home and into the vehicle and perhaps to stay with them at the medical facility. Many seniors feel more comfortable with someone from their congregation rather than with a paid outsider.

VETERANS SERVICES

Veterans and their spouses are eligible for a variety of services at reduced costs: burial in veterans cemeteries, adult day care, counseling, respite, nursing home care, prescription assistance, health care, and assisted living.

With all of the above services, assistance may not be available in every location. It is also important to remember that most elders want to stay as independent as possible. Be sensitive to the fact that accepting "government help" may be awkward or embarrassing to them.

Resources

■ Area Agency on Aging and Disability   (615) 255-1010

■ Aging & Disability Resource Center   1-877-973-6467

■ State Health Insurance Program   1-877-801-0044

■ Council on Aging *Directory of Services for Seniors*   (615) 353-4235
  (copies also available at public libraries)
  http://www.councilonaging-midtn.org

Resources
and
Inventories

General Resource List

1.	**AGING & DISABILITY RESOURCE CONNECTIONS**	**(615) 255-1010**
	Outside Metro Nashville	1 (877) 973-6467
	Call for information on a wide range of services for senior citizens in Middle Tennessee.	
2.	**COUNCIL ON AGING OF GREATER NASHVILLE**	**(615) 353-4235**
	Publishes the Directory of Services for Seniors that lists services for seniors in 13 counties of northern Middle Tennessee. The book is free for seniors and their families and is distributed at libraries in Cheatham, Davidson, Dickson, Houston, Humphreys, Montgomery, Robertson, Rutherford, Stewart, Sumner, Trousdale, Williamson, and Wilson Counties. The information in the printed Directory is also available on the web at: http://www.councilonaging-midtn.org	
3.	**ELDERCARE LOCATOR**	**1 (800) 677-1116**
	Toll-free help in identifying community resources for seniors nationwide. When calling, know the name and address of person you are assisting and the type of assistance needed.	
4.	**LEGAL AID SOCIETY OF MIDDLE TN AND THE CUMBERLANDS**	
	Clarksville office	**(931) 552-6656**
	Gallatin office	**(615) 451-1880**
	Murfreesboro office	**(615) 890-0905**
	Nashville office	**(615) 244-6610**
5.	**FORMS AND CHECKLISTS**	
	Downloadable forms are available on the website of the Council on Aging of Greater Nashville, www.councilonaging-midtn.org.	

SENIOR CENTERS *are also a good resource in each of the communities that they serve.*

Financial Records Inventories

Bank Accounts / Safe Deposit Box

BANK NAME	ACCOUNT #	ACCOUNT TYPE	NAMES / SIGNATURE AUTHORITY	VALUE
SAFE DEPOSIT BOX?		LOCATION:	Box #	
KEY LOCATED:			RENEWAL DATE:	
LIST OF BOX CONTENTS:				

Financial Records Inventories

Bank Account Automatic Deposits/Withdrawals

ACCOUNT	AMOUNT	DATE OF AUTO TRANSACTION	DEPOSIT OR WITHDRAWAL	PAYABLE TO	RECEIVED FROM

Financial Records Inventories

Investments: Stock, Mutual Funds, Partnerships

TYPE	BROKER / HOLDER	VALUE	ACCOUNT NAME	LOCATION OF CERTIFICATE

Financial Records Inventories

Real Estate Owned

INSURANCE POLICY LOCATED	LOCATION OF TITLE DOCUMENTS	TITLE IN NAME OF	MORTGAGE AMOUNT	ADDRESS

Financial Records Inventories

Personal Property (INCLUDE AUTOMOBILES, JEWELRY, ETC.)

TYPE	MAKE	MODEL	SERIAL / VIN #	VALUE	LOCATION

Financial Records Inventories

Liabilities: Credit Cards

NAME ON CARD	ISSUING BANK / COMPANY	ACCOUNT NUMBER	BALANCE

Financial Records Inventories

Mortgages and Other Debts

LENDER	ACOUNT NUMBER	BALANCE	PAYMENT AMOUNT	DUE DATE

Insurance Inventories

Life Insurance

POLICY LOCATED	INSURANCE COMPANY	TYPE / AMOUNT	POLICY NUMBER	BENEFICIARY(IES)	PREMIUM AMOUNT	DUE DATE

Insurance Inventories

Property/Casualty Insurance (including Automobile)

POLICY LOCATED	INSURANCE COMPANY	TYPE / AMOUNT	POLICY NUMBER	BENEFICIARY(IES)	PREMIUM AMOUNT	DUE DATE

Insurance Inventories

Health / Medical Insurance and Long term Care Insurance

POLICY LOCATED	INSURANCE COMPANY	TYPE / AMOUNT	POLICY NUMBER	BENEFICIARY(IES)	PREMIUM AMOUNT	DUE DATE

COUNCIL ON
AGING

Insurance Inventories

Burial Insurance / Prepaid Funeral

DUE DATE	PREMIUM AMOUNT	BENEFICIARY(IES)	POLICY NUMBER	TYPE / AMOUNT	INSURANCE COMPANY	POLICY LOCATED

Legal Inventory

Location of:	LAST WILL AND TESTAMENT	DURABLE POWER OF ATTORNEY	POWER OF ATTORNEY FOR HEALTH CARE (Appointment of Health Care Agent)	LIVING WILL (Advance Care Plan)	INCOME TAX RETURNS	MILITARY SERVICE DISCHARGE PAPERS (DD214)	MARRIAGE LICENSE	BURIAL PLOT CERTIFICATE

Medication Records Forms

SENIOR'S COPY

Medication Record Form

NAME:

NEXT OF KIN (Including Phone Number):

PRIMARY CARE PROVIDER (Including Phone Number):

OTHER PROVIDERS (Including Phone Numbers):

ALLERGIES TO MEDICATIONS OR FOOD:

PHARMACY (Including Phone Number):

MEDICATION NAME	DOSAGE	REASON TAKEN	TIME(S) OF DAY TAKEN	PRESCRIBING DOCOTR
EXAMPLE:				
NORVASC	10 mg	HIGH BLOOD PRESSURE	8:00 am	DR SMITH (Cardiologist)

Medication Records Forms

SENIOR'S COPY

Medication Record Form (CONT'D)

MEDICATION NAME	DOSAGE	REASON TAKEN	TIME(S) OF DAY TAKEN	PRESCRIBING DOCOTR

Medication Records Forms

CAREGIVER'S COPY

Medication Record Form

NAME:

NEXT OF KIN (Including Phone Number):

PRIMARY CARE PROVIDER (Including Phone Number):

OTHER PROVIDERS (Including Phone Numbers):

ALLERGIES TO MEDICATIONS OR FOOD:

PHARMACY (Including Phone Number):

MEDICATION NAME	DOSAGE	REASON TAKEN	TIME(S) OF DAY TAKEN	PRESCRIBING DOCOTR
EXAMPLE:				
NORVASC	10 mg	HIGH BLOOD PRESSURE	8:00 am	DR SMITH (Cardiologist)

Medication Records Forms

CAREGIVER'S COPY

Medication Record Form (CONT'D)

MEDICATION NAME	DOSAGE	REASON TAKEN	TIME(S) OF DAY TAKEN	PRESCRIBING DOCOTR

List of Current Medical Problems

List of Current Medical Problems

NAME:

NEXT OF KIN:

PHONE NUMBER:

MEDICAL PROBLEM	PROVIDER(S) YOU SEE FOR THIS (INCLUDING SPECIALTY)	PROVIDER'S PHONE NUMBER	DATES YOU LAST SAW THE PROVIDER ABOUT THIS ISSUE										
EXAMPLE:													
HIGH BLOOD PRESSURE	DR JOE SMITH	615-555-5555	AUGUST 10, 2004										

Glossary of Medical Conditions

Adenocarcinoma: Cancer that develops in the lining or inner surface of an organ.

Agnosia: The loss of ability to recognize people, objects, sounds, shapes, or smells.

Alzheimer's disease: A neurodegenerative brain disorder characterized by loss of memory, decision-making, aphasia, agnosia, and apraxia. It is the most common type of dementia.

Anticoagulant: Also known as a "blood thinner"; a medication that keeps blood from clotting.

Aphasia: The inability to speak or understand language which is due to brain damage or dementia.

Apraxia: The inability to carry out previously learned purposeful movements.

Arrhythmia: Abnormal heart rhythm.

Atherosclerosis: The building up of plaque in the inner lining of an artery.

Atrophy: A continuous muscle decline which follows a period of immobility or disuse.

Autoimmune disease: A process where the body's immune system attacks and destroys its own tissue that it mistakes for foreign matter.

Bradycardia: Abnormally slow heartbeat (less than 60 beats per minute).

Candidiasis: Also known as a yeast infection or thrush. A fungal infection caused by any of the Candida species.

Cerebrovascular accident (CVA): Also called a stroke. Caused by a lack of blood supply to the brain.

Cholecystitis: Inflammation of the gallbladder wall.

Chronic Obstructive Pulmonary Disorder: Also known as COPD. An umbrella term for lung diseases (emphysema, chronic bronchitis, and bronchiectasis) which are characterized by obstruction of airflow that interferes with normal breathing.

Claudication: Arm or leg pain due to a poor supply of oxygen to the muscles.

Dementia: A progressive, non-reversible decline in brain function that affects memory, language, attention, and problem solving. There are several types of dementia: Alzheimer's disease, vascular dementia, Pick's disease, and dementia with Lewy bodies.

Diverticulosis: Also known as diverticular disease. A condition that occurs when small pouches (diverticula) in the colon push outward through weak spots in the colon.

Eczema: Inflammation of the upper layers of skin that causes itching and sometimes crusting, scaling, or blisters.

Edema: Swelling of an organ or tissue due to the build-up of fluid.

Embolus: An object that migrates from one part of the body to another and causes blockage of a blood vessel.

Gastroesophageal reflux disease: Also known as GERD. Chronic problems of heartburn, difficulty swallowing, and sometimes chest pain caused by abnormal reflux of gastric contents into the esophagus.

Heart failure: A condition in which the heart is unable to fill with or pump an adequate amount of blood through the body. This condition can result from any structural or functional cardiac disorder.

Impaction: Trapping of hardened stool in the rectum.

Ischemic heart disease: Coronary artery disease or coronary heart disease caused by narrowing of the coronary arteries and decreased blood flow to the heart.

Incontinence: A lack of voluntary control of one's bowels or urine.

Myocardial infarction: (A heart attack). Occurs when blood supply to one or more regions of the heart muscle is interrupted, resulting in lack of oxygen supply and death of heart tissue.

Parkinson's disease: A degenerative disorder of the central nervous system characterized by muscle rigidity, tremor, and slowing of physical movements. Motor skills and speech are often impaired.

Syncope: Fainting caused by insufficient blood supply to the brain.

Thrombus: Also known as a blood clot.

Transient ischemic attack (TIA): Many times referred to as a mini stroke. The event is caused by a temporary disturbance of blood supply to the brain. Stroke-like symptoms occur for less than 24 hours.

Varicose vein: An abnormally dilated vein, usually found in the legs.

Glossary of Medical Tests, Therapies & Procedures

Adjuvant therapy: Treatment that is used in combination with other therapies to maximize effectiveness. Examples: radiation, chemotherapy, and hormone therapy.

Computed tomography: (CT or CAT scan) A medical imaging method that takes cross-sectional images of the brain or other internal organs done to detect any abnormalities. The scanner is a large square machine with a hole in the middle. The patient lies still on a table that is inserted into the machine. The test lasts 5-30 minutes.

Debridement: Removal of dead, damaged, or infected tissue from a wound or burn. Removal can be surgical, mechanical, or autolytic.

Defibrillator: An electronic device used to establish normal heartbeat by delivering electric shock. This is often used when professionals are doing CPR on a patient.

Dual energy x-ray absorptiometry (DEXA): Imaging technique that uses a very low dose of radiation to measure bone density for the diagnosis of osteoporosis.

Echocardiogram: An ultrasound of the heart that can visualize and assess heart valves, abnormal communication between the right and left sides of the heart, the volume of blood being pumped through the heart, and ejection fraction.

Ejection fraction: The measurement of the blood pumped out of the ventricles of the heart. An echocardiogram measures the ejection fraction.

Electrocardiogram (ECG or EKG): A test that records the electrical activity of the heart, shows abnormal rhythms, and detects damage to the heart muscle.

Laminectomy: A surgical procedure including removal of a portion of the lamina to provide more room in the vertebral canal. This is usually performed to treat disc herniation or spinal canal stenosis.

Magnetic resonance imaging (MRI): A diagnostic test that produces a two-dimensional view of an internal organ. The patient is placed on a table that slides into the scanning machine and is required to remain still through the test, which lasts 15 to 45 minutes.

Occupational Therapy (OT): Treatment to help individuals develop, relearn, or maintain the skills needed to participate in all areas of life. Occupational therapists help patients with fine motor skills as well as hand-eye coordination.

Physical Therapy (PT): Treatment utilizing physical activities and exercises to condition muscles and restore strength and movement. The health care provider may order this after a patient has had an injury or an illness.

Recreational Therapy (RT): Treatment used by therapists to improve or maintain physical, mental, and emotional well-being. These treatments can include arts and crafts, animals, music, drama, and games.

Speech Therapy (ST): Treatment to correct swallowing or communication problems. Therapists may utilize physical strengthening and memory exercises as well as the use of communication aides.

Thallium stress test: A type of nuclear scanning test which shows how well blood flows to the heart muscle.

Transesophageal echocardiography (TEE): An invasive procedure during which an ultrasound of the heart is taken by inserting a specialized probe into one's esophagus.

COMMON BLOOD TESTS

Blood cultures: In this blood test, a culture of the blood is taken to determine if infection is spreading through the blood stream. The culture will help identify what bacteria are in a patient's blood to help the physician determine the correct antibiotic to prescribe. Final results of the blood culture are generally available in three days.

BMP (Basic Metabolic Panel): This blood chemistry test is ordered to determine if electrolytes within the body are in balance, if the kidneys are functioning properly, and if the blood glucose level is within normal limits.

CBC (Complete blood count): This blood test gives information about the cells in the blood. The cells are generally divided into three types: white blood cells, red blood cells, and platelets. Although a CBC is ordered for many different reasons, it is commonly ordered if the healthcare provider thinks a patient may have anemia or an infection.

Erythrocyte Sedimentation Rate: Also known as "ESR" or "sed rate." This blood test measures inflammation within the body. Although it does not indicate where the inflammation is present in the body, it is useful to diagnose temporal arteritis and polymyalgia rheumatica.

TSH (Thyroid stimulating hormone): This test is often ordered in combination with a thyroid hormone level test ("T4"). Together, these blood tests are ordered if it is suspected that the patient's thyroid is either overactive (hyperthyroidism) or underactive (hypothyroidism).

Urinalysis: Also known as a "UA," this test detects many things that may be present in a patient's urine (including red and white blood cells, glucose, and protein). It may be ordered to see if there are bacteria causing a urinary tract infection. Many times a **culture and sensitivity** (C&S) is also ordered. The C&S will identify the bacteria causing the infection and help the physician determine the correct antibiotic to prescribe.

Future Caregiving Checklist

Future Caregiving Checklist

WHAT WILL BE NEEDED?	WHO WILL BE RESPONSIBLE?	HOW WILL IT BE PAID FOR?	NOW WHAT? BACK-UP PLAN
DAILY LIVING ACTIVITIES			
Nutrition: Menu planning, buying food, cooking, serving, cleaning up			
Hygiene: Bathing, shaving, toileting, buying supplies			
Housekeeping			
Clothing: Shopping, selecting, cleaning, mending			
Recreation: Social activities, friends, clubs, sports, exercise			
Transportation: work, social, medical, emergency			
Religious activities			
Vacations, holiday trips			
HEALTH & MEDICAL			
Exams: doctor, dentist, specialists			
Medicine: refills, administration, monitoring effects			
Emergencies: transportation, paperwork			
Special treatments, adaptive equipment			

Future Caregiving Checklist

Future Caregiving Checklist

WHAT WILL BE NEEDED?	WHO WILL BE RESPONSIBLE?	HOW WILL IT BE PAID FOR?	NOW WHAT? BACK-UP PLAN
HEALTH & MEDICAL (Cont'd)			
Mental Health needs			
Emergencies: transportation, paperwork			
Special treatments, adaptive equipment			
Mental Health needs			
RESIDENTIAL			
Monitoring: Unannounced visits, visiting, problem-solving, annual review, oversee changes in residence			
ADMINISTRATIVE / LEGAL			
Conservator or Representative Payee or Responsible Party			
Monitor all service providers			
Maintain written records			
Communicate with family members			
Advance Directives: Will, Trust, Power of Attorney, Power of Attorney for Health Care, Living Will, Letters of Direction			

Questions to Ask When Hiring a Private Care Service

- May I contact others who have used this service?

- What is your philosophy of care? What is your mission statement?

- What type of family caregiver support do you offer?

- Why should I use you over another agency?

- Do you set up and identify a clear plan of care? If so, how is this set up and what does it include? How do we communicate and modify as care needs change?

- What happens in the event a caregiver is ill or doesn't show up for work?

- What happens if I need to reach you outside normal business hours?

- Does the same caregiver come each time?

- What happens if a caregiver is not a "good fit" for my loved one?

- What do you look for in employees? How would you support them in their caring for my loved one?

- How do you bill?

- Am I required to sign a contract?

- Do you have workman's compensation benefits and liability insurance? May I see your Certificate of Insurance?

- What about other issues such as TB skin tests, CPR training, etc.?

- Tell me about criminal background checks on your employees. Do they cover checking nurse abuse registries? Do they check Tennessee records only or records in all states of residence for the last ten years?

- Do you conduct pre-employment or scheduled random drug screens on your employees?

- In addition to your business license, are you licensed in this state as a Personal Support Service Agency?

Recipes for Additional Nutrition

CALORIE AND PROTEIN BOOSTERS – EASY WAYS TO ADD EXTRA NUTRITION

Powdered Milk – Add 2-4 tablespoons of the dry powder to 1 cup of milk. Mix into puddings, potatoes, soups, and cooked cereals. Contains 33 calories and 3 grams of protein for each tablespoon.

Eggs – Add to casseroles, meatloaf, mashed potatoes, creamed dishes, pancake batter, and French toast. Add chopped boiled eggs to many foods. Never use raw eggs in uncooked foods. Each egg provides 80 calories and 7 grams protein.

Butter or Margarine – Add to casseroles, sandwiches, vegetables, cooked cereals, breads, and muffins. Each teaspoon provides 45 calories.

Cheeses – Give as snacks or on sandwiches. Add to casseroles, potatoes, eggs, and vegetables. Cheese provides 100 calories and 7 grams of protein per ounce.

Wheat Germ – Add 1-2 tablespoons to cereals. Mix into meat dishes, cookie batter, and casseroles. Each tablespoon contains 25 calories and also adds fiber.

Mayonnaise or Salad Dressings – Use extra on sandwiches, in salads, as a raw vegetable dip, or in sauces for vegetables. Contains 45 calories per teaspoon.

Evaporated Milk – Use in place of whole milk, in desserts, baked good, meat dishes, and cooked cereals. Contains 25 calories and 1 gram of protein for each tablespoon.

Sour Cream – Add to potatoes, casseroles, dips, sauces, and baked goods. Contains 25 calories for each tablespoon.

Sweetened Condensed Milk – Add to pies, puddings, or milkshakes. Contains 60 calories and 1 gram of protein for each tablespoon.

Peanut Butter – Serve on toast, crackers, bananas, apples, or celery or add to puddings. Contains 95 calories and 4 grams of protein per tablespoon.

Instant breakfast drinks – Add to milk and milkshakes. The dry powder packet contains 130 calories and 7 grams of protein. When mixed with 8 ounces of whole milk, the total calories and protein are essentially the same as many commercial supplements.

Gravies – Use liberally on mashed potatoes, meats, and bread.

Recipes for Additional Nutrition

MILKSHAKE RECIPES

*Commercial supplements are convenient for many families. However, if cost is an issue, there are less expensive alternatives that can be made at home which provide similar nutritional content. When egg substitute is included, this refers to frozen egg substitutes found in the grocery stores. Remember; **never** use raw eggs in foods that will not be cooked before being eaten. People with an allergy to eggs should not use the egg substitute since it contains egg whites. A couple of examples might be:*

Apple-Cinnamon Shake	Lemon Shake
1 cup apple pie filling 1 cup vanilla ice cream ½ cup whole milk Dash of cinnamon Blend together in a blender.	½ - 2 cups of vanilla ice cream ½ cup of lemonade concentrate (frozen) ½ cup buttermilk ¼ cup egg substitute (if desired) Blend together in a blender.
Basic Milkshake	**Peach Shake**
1 cup ice cream ½ cup of half and half ¼ cup of egg substitute (if desired) 2 tablespoons sugar (optional) Blend together in a blender.	1 cup whole milk 1 cup canned peaches 1 cup vanilla ice cream ¼ teaspoon salt ¼ teaspoon vanilla Blend together in a blender.
Chocolate-Peanut Butter Shake	**Sherbet Shake**
½ cup of half and half 3 tablespoons of creamy peanut butter 3 tablespoons chocolate syrup 1 ½ cups of chocolate or vanilla ice cream Blend together in a blender.	1 cup sherbet (orange is great) ¼ - ½ cup of whipping cream 1-2 tablespoons of corn syrup Blend together in a blender.
Lemon Cream Freeze	**Strawberry Fruit Shake**
½ - 1 cup fruit yogurt (lemon) ¼ cup half and half ½ cup cottage cheese 1 package instant breakfast drink mix Add sugar, if desired Blend and freeze.	2 cups frozen strawberries ½ cup crushed pineapple ½ cup water ½ medium banana 6 tablespoons sugar ¼ cup lemon juice 2 tablespoons honey Blend together in a blender.

Special diet restrictions need to be considered with any of the suggestions provided. Some restrictions may apply to individuals. Always have guidance from your physician or registered dietitian if there are questions.

~ Notes ~

_____

_____

_____

_____

_____

_____

_____

_____

_____

_____

_____

_____

_____

_____

_____

_____

_____

_____

_____

_____

_____

_____

Notes

_____

_____

_____

_____

_____

_____

_____

_____

_____

_____

_____

_____

_____

_____

_____

_____

_____

_____

_____

_____

_____

_____

~ Notes ~

CPSIA information can be obtained at www.ICGtesting.com
Printed in the USA
LVOW121450210911

247249LV00001B/2/P